MCQs in Travel Medicine

MCQs in Travel Medicine

Dom Colbert MD, BSc, FRCSI, CTH™, FFTM (Glasg), FCS (ECSA)

Department of International Health and Tropical Medicine,
Royal College of Surgeons, Ireland, Travel Medicine Society of Ireland,
College of Surgeons of East, Central and Southern Africa,
National University of Ireland, Galway

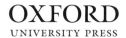

OXFORD
UNIVERSITY PRESS

Great Clarendon Street, Oxford, OX2 6DP,
United Kingdom

Oxford University Press is a department of the University of Oxford.
It furthers the University's objective of excellence in research, scholarship,
and education by publishing worldwide. Oxford is a registered trade mark of
Oxford University Press in the UK and in certain other countries

© Oxford University Press, 2013

The moral rights of the authors have been asserted

British Library Cataloguing in Publication Data

Data available

ISBN 978-0-19-966452-8

Printed and bound by
CPI Group (UK) Ltd, Croydon, CR0 4YY

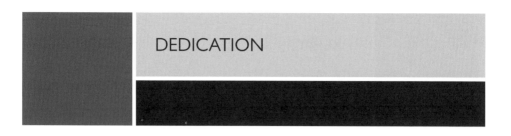

DEDICATION

For a new generation of travellers, my grandchildren,
Dominic, Gino, Conor, Lily, Patrick, Danielle, Robert, Helena

The Author's royalties from this book are donated to AboutFace, a UK-based organization of
volunteer surgeons, who travel to India each year to correct facial deformities in
those who cannot afford such surgery.

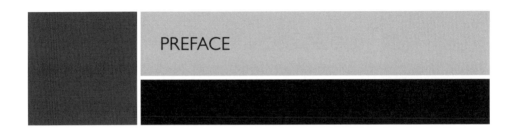

PREFACE

Travel health has expanded enormously in recent times, with over 2 billion people on the move every year. Such an expansion has brought on medical problems on a scale never before encountered, but which are now a daily challenge. Thus we are faced with preparing people of all ages, and sometimes those with indifferent health, to travel to places where strange and exotic diseases exist. Equally we are faced with the problems they bring back home.

In addition to this, globalization has brought massive demographic changes, particularly in developed countries, so that 'new' populations and 'new' diseases, many of which were previously unheard of, are present at our clinics and hospitals. All this is compounded by global warming, which is allowing a variety of tropical diseases, in particular arthropod-borne diseases such as West Nile fever and dengue fever, to creep north and south from the equator into Europe, Asia, the USA, and Australia.

This book addresses these problems in a practical way by challenging the reader over a wide range of topics. It encompasses the whole range of travel medicine from simple entomology to problems found in the returned traveller. Although I set out to write a short MCQ book for those preparing for exams in travel medicine, I finished by writing a small textbook of travel medicine in MCQ format. Because of this I hope the book will be of value to anyone working in travel medicine whether doctor, nurse, pharmacist, or interested healthcare worker. I also had in mind those who are responsible for the health of our growing immigrant population or who plan to work overseas, especially in the tropics.

The book is designed to be easy to use. It contains almost 800 questions, each with four options as answers, only one of which is correct or is considered the best. The detailed explanations are meant to teach and challenge the reader, who is finally asked to do a self-test in chapter 19.

I recognize that everyone in health care is extremely busy and has little time to spare for professional reading. However, it is my hope that the division of this book into many sub-sections will allow for a pick-up, put-down approach, in which even a 10-minute session will be beneficial. Most of all, I hope the reader will enjoy this work and share some of the excitement and thrill of exploring a fascinating and expanding field of medicine.

As ever I am happy to receive and incorporate constructive comments, suggestions, and corrections from any reader.

I acknowledge the patience of my wife Doreen, who has endured the never-ending vagaries of a doctor's life. I also acknowledge the professional advice of Nicola Wilson and Caroline Smith from OUP and the painstaking editorial direction of Dr Lesley Montford from Anglosphere Editing. In a special way I am indebted to my friend and distinguished colleague Dr Gerard Flaherty of the Galway Medical School, who has been so generous with his time and so sound in his advice.

Dom Colbert
Galway 2012

CONTENTS

ABBREVIATIONS

ACT	artemisinin combined treatment
ADE	antibody-dependent enhancement
AGE	arterial gas embolism
AMS	acute mountain sickness
anti-HBcAg	anti-hepatitis B core antigen
anti-HBs	hepatitis B surface antibody
AP	atovaquone 250 mg/proguanil 100 mg
ARI	acute respiratory infection
ART	anti-retroviral therapy
AS	acute strongyloidosis
ATBF	African tick bite fever
BCG	Bacille Calmette-Guerin
BCR	benefit–cost ratio
BSS	bismuth subsalicylate
BTI	*Bacillus thuringiensis* Israeli
CABG	coronary artery bypass graft
CAP	community-acquired pneumonia
CBF	cerebral blood flow
CCF	chronic congestive heart failure
CDC	Centres for Disease Control and Prevention
CFS	chronic fatigue syndrome
CFU	colony-forming unit
CL	cutaneous leishmaniasis
CLM	*Cutaneous larva migrans*
CNS	central nervous system
CPRV	chromatographically purified rabies vaccine
CRFM	chloroquine-resistant falciparum malaria
CRP	C reactive protein
CSF	cerebrospinal fluid
CVA	cerebrovascular accident
CXR	chest X-ray

DC	dendritic cells
DEAC	diffusely enteroadherent *E. coli*
DEC	diethylcarbamazine
DEET	diethyltoluamide
DHA	dihydroartemisinin
DHF	dengue haemorrhagic fever
DOTS	directly observed therapy strategy
DV	dengue virus
DVT	deep venous thrombosis
ECS	environmental control systems
EHEC	enterohaemorrhagic *E. coli*
EIEC	enteroinvasive *E. coli*
EM	eosinophilic meningitis
ENL	erythema nodosum leprosum
ES	exposure to symptoms
ESR	erythrocyte sedimentation rate
ETEC	enterotoxigenic *E. coli*
FQ	fluoroquinolones
G6PD	glucose 6-phosphate dehydrogenase
GCS	graduated compression stockings
HAART	highly active anti-retroviral treatment
HACE	high-altitude cerebral oedema
HAPE	high-altitude pulmonary oedema
HAT	human African trypanosomiasis
HAV	hepatitis A virus
HBV	hepatitis B virus
HBeAg	hepatitis B e-antigen
HBsAg	hepatitis B surface antigen
HCT	hypoxic challenge test
HDCV	human diploid cell vaccine
HEPA	high-efficiency particle air filtration
HIG	modern human immunoglobulin
HUS	haemolytic uremic syndrome
HRP-2	histidine-rich protein-2 antigen
ICP	intracranial pressure
ICT	immunochromatography
ID	intradermal
IFAT	indirect immunofluorescence antibody test
ILI	influenza-like illness

IM	intramuscular
INH	isoniazid
IPV	inactivated parenteral polio vaccine
ISTM	International Society of Travel Medicine
KCV	killed cholera vaccine
LF	lymphatic filariasis
MCV4	meningococcal conjugate vaccine
MDRTB	multidrug-resistant TB
MI	myocardial infarction
ML	mucocutaneous leishmaniasis
MS	multiple sclerosis
MVA	motor vehicle accident
MVP	mitral valve prolapse
NCC	neurocysticercosis
NNT	number of persons needed to treat
NPP	neuropsychiatric problems
NWCL	New World cutaneous leishmaniasis
OC	oral contraceptive
OCP	Oncocerciasis Control Program
OCV	oral cholera vaccine
OPSS	overwhelming post-splenectomy sepsis
OPV	oral poliomyelitis vaccine
ORS	oral rehydration solution
OTC	over the counter
OWCL	Old World cutaneous leishmaniasis
PABA	*para*-aminobenzoic acid
PAM	primary amoebic meningoencephalitis
PaO$_2$	pressure of oxygen in arterial blood
PCEV	purified chick embryo vaccine
PCR	polymerase chain reaction
PDEV	purified duck embryo vaccine
PEP	post-exposure prophylaxis
PKDL	post Kala-azar dermal leishmaniasis
pLDH	plasmodium lactate dehydrogenase
PoEP	post-exposure prophylaxis
POPS	pulmonary overpressurization syndrome
PPD	purified protein derivative
PQP	piperaquine
PreEp	pre-exposure prophylaxis

PTS	post-traumatic stress
PUO	pyrexia of unknown origin
PVRV	purified vero cell rabies vaccine
PZQ	praziquantel
REAO	rapid epidemiological assessment for onchocerciasis
RDT	rapid diagnostic test
RIG	rabies immune globulin
RRR	reporting rate ratio
SADS	sudden adult death syndrome
SAT	serum agglutination test
SBET	standby emergency treatment
SC	subcutaneous
SCUBA	self-contained underwater breathing apparatus
SIDS	sudden infant death syndrome
SPF	skin protection factor
SR	slow release
STEC	shiga-toxin-producing *E. coli*
STI	sexually transmitted infection
TD	travellers' diarrhoea
TMP-SMX	trimethoprim-sulfamethoxazole
TNF-α	tumour necrosis factor-α
TOCP	tri-ortho-cresylphosphate
TPE	tropical pulmonary eosinophilia
TQS	tetanus quick sticks
TT	tuberculin test
URI	upper respiratory infection
UV	ultraviolet
VAPP	vaccine-associated paralytic poliomyelitis
VFRs	visiting friends and relatives
VHF	viral haemorrhagic fever
VGIG	varicella zoster immune globulin
Vi	parenteral typhoid vaccine
VL	visceral leishmaniasis
VOCs	volatile organic compounds
VTE	venous thromboembolism
WHO	World Health Organization
WNV	West Nile virus
YFVA-ND	yellow fever vaccine-associated neurotropic disease
YFVA-VD	yellow fever vaccine-associated viscerotropic disease

Setting up a travel medical service involves time, money, patience, and continual updating of information. Ultimately such a service cannot be viable unless there is a sufficient throughput of patients to warrant its existence. It is likely that in a multipractice clinic one practitioner will be very interested in travel medicine. Other members of the group should refer all travellers to him or her. In many countries, particularly in the UK, the practice nurse is the one who does most pre-travel consultations. However, this should be a shared responsibility between nurse and doctor so that maximum benefit is provided for both the patient and the clinic.

1. **General considerations about travel clinics**
   A. Most general practices are suitably prepared to run a travel clinic service
   B. A refrigerator dedicated solely to vaccine storage is a most important physical item in a travel clinic
   C. More than 20 patients per week are needed to warrant setting up a travel clinic
   D. At least two people, e.g. doctor and nurse, are needed to run a travel clinic

2. **Which of the following do you consider to be the most important thing for the travel medical practitioner to have?**
   A. Membership of a travel medical society
   B. Access to internet services
   C. A textbook of travel medicine
   D. A textbook of tropical medicine

3. **Which of the following is the most important thing for a travel clinic to do?**
   A. Keep permanent medical records
   B. Have all travel-related vaccines available
   C. Be familiar with the destination of the traveller
   D. Provide a pre-consultation form detailing all facts relevant to a particular traveller and the proposed itinerary

4. Which of these would you consider to be the most common problem when managing a travel clinic?

A. Out-of-date vaccines

B. Adverse reactions to vaccines

C. The traveller dictating which vaccines are needed for his or her travel

D. Insufficient time to give to individual travellers

1. B. This is the preferred option from the above. A vaccine-dedicated fridge is essential, with the temperature kept between 2 and 8°C, ideally at 5°C. A maximum/minimum thermometer should be used to monitor this. Vaccines should not be stored in the door compartments.

Where vaccines are freeze-stored, e.g. varicella in North America, the temperature should be kept around −200°C. Records of vaccines stored and their expiry dates should be meticulously kept.

Most family practices are not suitable to set themselves up as specialist travel clinics unless the expertise of those running them, the equipment needed, and the throughput of patients is satisfactory. While the majority of practices deal with fewer than 20 travellers per week, many consider that 10 per week is the minimum needed to warrant such a practice.

2. B. All of the above are important, but internet access to the best current medical practice in travel medicine is essential. There are numerous sites that provide this information and also give reports of current outbreaks of disease overseas. Everyone has free access to the WHO and CDC sites but there are other excellent sites dedicated to travel medicine for which a fee is payable, e.g. Travax. Lists of these sites are readily available from any local society, from the International Society of Travel Medicine (ISTM.org) or can be found in any textbook of travel medicine.

3. A. Retention of permanent records is essential. Such records will contain travellers' itineraries, activities, medical history, immunization history, and subsequent follow-up. Keeping records in this way allows information to be transmitted years later to the subject or to other healthcare providers in other locations or in other countries. It is also necessary for insurance purposes should the need arise. Clearly the other options listed are important but not essential.

4. D. Each pre-travel consultation takes time, patience, and space. It takes a minimum of 20 minutes to complete an average consultation and much longer depending on the patient's age, health status, intended activities, length of trip, time of year and location of the proposed travel. In addition to the other options listed the following present problems: last-minute consultations, phone calls for advice, need for up-to-date information for clinic personnel, conflicting advice from different sources, cost of vaccines (especially for family groups visiting friends and relatives), language difficulties, and vague itineraries.

chapter

2

EPIDEMIOLOGICAL AND GEOGRAPHICAL CONSIDERATIONS

QUESTIONS

It is useful to have a good knowledge of geography and to have at least a globe or atlas in the clinic so that the patient can point out a planned itinerary. Appropriate internet facilities must be available so that information on local diseases, current outbreaks, and required immunizations can be accessed speedily.

1. **Which of the following infects the largest number of people worldwide?**
   A. Schistosomiasis
   B. Trypanosomiasis
   C. Amoebiasis
   D. Filariasis

2. **The likelihood of a traveller becoming ill is greatest in**
   A. India
   B. Thailand
   C. South Africa
   D. Argentina

3. **Which of these species is the most common cause of clinical disease worldwide?**
   A. *Brucella abortus*
   B. *Brucella melitensis*
   C. *Brucella suis*
   D. *Brucella canis*

4. **Mortality from malaria has only been documented in**
   A. *P. falciparum*, *P. malariae*, and *P. knowlesi* infections
   B. *P. falciparum* and *P. vivax* infections
   C. *P. falciparum* and *P. ovale* infections
   D. All five types

5. **Lassa fever is named after a town in**
   A. Nigeria
   B. South Africa
   C. China
   D. South America

6. Which species of malaria is confined almost exclusively to West Africa?

A. *P. falciparum*

B. *P. malaria*

C. *P. ovale*

D. *P. vivax*

7. Endemic falciparum malaria is still found in

A. The Dominican Republic

B. Taiwan

C. Brunei

D. The Maldives

8. *Plasmodium knowlesi*

A. Is indistinguishable microscopically from *P. falciparum*

B. Is almost always clinically similar to a *P. falciparum* infection

C. Responds well to chloroquine

D. Is most common in West Africa

9. The incidence of typhoid fever is highest in

A. India

B. Mexico

C. Indonesia

D. Mozambique

10. The infective dose of *S. typhi* is estimated at

A. One organism

B. 1000 organisms

C. 100,000 organisms

D. More than a million organisms

11. To eliminate the risk from ingested *S. typhi*

A. Heat water and food to 60°C

B. Keep food in the deep freeze (–21°C)

C. Store all meat and dairy products in the fridge

D. Treat all sewage in accordance with current regulations

12. *S. typhi* is most often spread to travellers apart from those visiting friends and relatives (VFRs) by

A. Droplet infection

B. Carriage by flies to food

C. Carriage in faeces of small mammals

D. Consumption of duck eggs

13. The risk of contracting falciparum malaria is greatest
A. On the Kenyan coast
B. In Kinshasa
C. In the island resorts off Thailand
D. In Nairobi

14. Cholera is still officially reported in
A. Fewer than five countries
B. Fewer than 10 countries
C. Fewer than 20 countries
D. Fewer than 100 countries

15. The most common way travellers contract leptospirosis is from
A. White-water river rafting
B. Ingesting leptospiral-contaminated food
C. Contact with farm animals
D. Hotel swimming pools

16. The most common cause of febrile jaundice in the traveller is
A. Malaria
B. Dengue fever
C. Acute viral hepatitis
D. Leptospirosis (Weil's disease)

17. Where is the traveller most likely to contract African tick bite fever (ATBF)?
A. Southern Africa
B. Kenya
C. Ethiopia
D. West Africa

18. Apart from the required immunizations and advice, anyone planning to go on daytime safaris in Tanzania, Kenya, or Uganda should be specifically warned of the danger of contracting
A. Yellow fever
B. Malaria
C. Human African trypanosomiasis (HAT)
D. Pulmonary histoplasmosis

19. Which of the following is associated with being bitten mainly during the darker hours?
A. Yellow fever
B. Dengue fever
C. African trypanosomiasis (sleeping sickness)
D. American trypanosomiasis (Chagas disease)

20. **Match the vector with the disease. Vector options may be used once, more than once, or not at all**

A. Malaria	1. Sandflies
B. Yellow fever	2. Mosquito
C. Leishmania	3. Tsetse fly
D. Loa loa	4. Flea
E. Dengue fever	5. Red fly (chrysops fly)
F. Onchocerciasis	6. Black fly (*Simulium damnosum*)

21. **Make the best matches for the following locations using options once, more than once, or not at all.**

A. South-East Asia	1. Giardiasis
B. Nepal	2. Espundia
C. South America	3. Altitude sickness
D. Russia	4. Campylobacter

22. **The most common cause of sore throat in the long-term visitor to tropical and subtropical regions is**

A. Viral or bacterial pharyngitis (as found in temperate climates)
B. Diphtheria
C. Acute HIV
D. One of the viral hemorrhagic fevers

23. **Chlorination as used widely in swimming pools fails to destroy**

A. *S. typhi*
B. Rotavirus
C. Giardial cysts
D. *E. coli*

24. **Match the diseases listed with the vectors that carry them. Options may be used once, more than once, or not at all**

A. Typhus	1. Mosquitoes
B. Cutaneous leishmaniasis	2. Ticks
C. West Nile fever	3. Fleas
D. Hantavirus	4. Sandflies

25. **Match the diseases listed with the vectors that carry them. Options may be used once, more than once, or not at all**

A. Lyme disease	1. Mosquito
B. Schistosomiasis	2. Black fly
C. River blindness	3. Ticks
D. Rabies	4. Aquatic snails
	5. Bats

26. Match the diseases listed with the vectors that carry them. Options may be used once, more than once, or not at all

A. Relapsing fever (borreliosis)   1. Lice
B. Chagas disease   2. Mosquitoes
C. Yellow fever   3. Triatomine bugs
D. Dengue fever   4. Ticks

27. Which causes the greatest number of deaths in humans?

A. Sharks
B. Crocodiles
C. Venomous snakes
D. Lions

28. Bear attacks have been reported from

A. Morocco
B. Nepal
C. Australia
D. Argentina

29. Which of these conditions is most common in urban areas?

A. Chagas disease
B. Bartonella
C. Dengue fever
D. Japanese encephalitis

30. Match the following regions with their comparative rates of homicide

A. Western Europe   1. Highest rate
B. Honduras   2. Second highest rate
C. Uganda   3. Third highest rate
D. USA   4. Fourth highest rate

31. Which of these diseases is currently notifable to the World Health Organization (WHO)?

A. Typhus
B. Cholera
C. HIV
D. Tuberculosis

32. Crude rates refer to rates calculated with

A. The total population of an area as the denominator
B. A specific age group as the denominator
C. A specific gender as the denominator
D. On the basis of small random samples in an area

33. **Infant mortality refers to the number of deaths of live infants when death occurs in the first**

A. 28 days of life
B. 3 months of life
C. 6 months of life
D. 12 months of life

34. **If 25 of 100 returned travellers present with travellers' diarrhoea (TD) you can say**

A. The prevalence of TD in that group is 25%
B. The incidence of TD in that group is 25%
C. The attack rate for TD in that group is 25%
D. All of the above are true

35. **Which of the following has the highest financial benefit–cost ratio (BCR) for travellers to East Africa?**

A. Chloroquine
B. Doxycycline
C. Proguanil
D. Fansidar

36. **Which of these vaccines has the highest BCR for the general traveller?**

A. Rabies
B. Typhoid
C. Hepatitis B
D. Hepatitis A

37. **The relationship between incidence rate, prevalence rate, and average duration of a communicable illness can be expressed by**

A. Incidence × prevalence = duration
B. Incidence × duration = prevalence
C. Incidence/duration = prevalence
D. Prevalence/duration = incidence

38. **The most common cause of serious arthropod-borne imported disease in travellers worldwide is**

A. Dengue fever
B. Tick typhus
C. Malaria
D. Japanese encephalitis

39. The most common cause of death from arthropod-borne imported disease in travellers worldwide is

A. Dengue fever

B. Tick typhus

C. Malaria

D. Japanese encephalitis

40. Where is the risk of *P. falciparum* infection greatest?

A. Thai–Myanmar border

B. West Africa

C. Assam

D. Cambodia

41. A non-immune traveller is most likely to contract yellow fever in

A. The Ivory coast

B. Peru

C. Mozambique

D. The Serengeti

42. Towns and cities in the 'yellow fever belt' are considered free from the danger of yellow fever if the proportion of houses around which breeding places exist for *Aedes aegypti* (aedes index) is less than

A. 20.0%

B. 10.0%

C. 1.0 %

D. 0.5%

43. The Centres for Disease Control and Prevention (CDC) has warned of current endemic yellow feve in which one of the following countries?

A. Argentina

B. Tunisia

C. The Maldives

D. Macao

44. The most common cause of *fatal injury* in travellers is

A. Motor vehicle accident (MVA)

B. Drowning

C. Falling, e.g. falls on land, climbing and skiing falls, sport-related falls

D. Mugging

45. The most common cause of *non-fatal injury* is

A. MVA

B. Drowning

C. Falling, e.g. falls on land, climbing and skiing falls, sport-related falls

D. Mugging

46. Estimated global incidence rates for TB are greatest in

  A. Sub-Saharan Africa

  B. India

  C. Eastern Europe

  D. South-East Asia

47. Which of the following do you consider has contributed most to the cure of TB in recent times?

  A. Streptomycin

  B. Correctly performed DOTS (directly observed therapy strategy)

  C. Poverty control

  D. Early diagnosis

48. What is the current major reservoir for avian flu H5N1?

  A. Wild ducks

  B. Jays and crows

  C. Rats

  D. Chickens

49. Lyme disease is

  A. Confined to the north-east of the USA

  B. Limited to parts of North America and Western Europe

  C. Found in temperate zones of the northern hemisphere

  D. Found in temperate zones in both northern and southern hemispheres

50. The insecticide of most use in the Oncocerciasis Control Program (OCP) is

  A. Permethrin

  B. DEET

  C. Temepos (abate)

  D. DDT

51. *Onchocerca volvulus*

  A. Is transmitted by the housefly

  B. Is transmitted by rodents

  C. Is confined to West Africa

  D. Has symptoms and signs in humans that are related to dead microfilariae

52. The usual way of determining the level of onchocerciasis in a poor rural community is to

  A. Count the palpable nodules

  B. Show that >80% of nodules contain *O. volvulus*

  C. Demonstrate microfilariae in skin and/or conjunctival snips

  D. Use serological tests

53. Where are you most likely to acquire schistosomiasis?

A. The Mekong delta

B. The Nile south of Luxor

C. The Zambezi near Victoria Falls

D. In the deeper reaches of the Amazon

54. Match the country with its predominant type(s) of schistosomiasis. Options may be used once, more than once, or not at all

A. Brazil   1. *S. hematobium*

B. Philippines   2. *S. mansoni*

C. Southern China   3. *S. japonicum*

D. Vietnam   4. *S. intercalatum*

E. Mozambique   5. *S. mekongi*

55. Which of the following is the leading cause of death from infectious disease in developing countries in all age groups?

A. Acute respiratory infection (ARI)

B. AIDS

C. Diarrhoeal diseases

D. Malaria

56. Which of the following is the leading cause of death from infectious disease in developing countries in under-five-year olds?

A. Diarrhoeal diseases

B. TB

C. Malaria

D. Measles

57. Where is the incidence of visceral leishmaniasis (VL) greatest?

A. Indian sub-continent

B. Sub-Saharan Africa

C. North Africa

D. Middle East

58. Parenteral transmission is most likely to occur with

A. Leishmaniasis

B. Hepatitis A

C. Blastocystis hominis

D. Varicella

59. The epidemiological pattern of dengue virus (DV) has shown

A. A steady decline in most dengue endemic regions since 1990

B. That outbreaks occur wherever *Ae. Aegypti* is found

C. A spread to many subtropical areas in recent times

D. A high incidence of dengue fever in sub-Saharan Africa

60. Tick-borne encephalitis (TBE)

A. Has reduced dramatically in incidence in the past 10 years

B. Has been eliminated from Siberia

C. Has no reporting system

D. Is now found in Norway

1. A. The three most common parasitic diseases worldwide, in order of frequency, are malaria, schistosomiasis, and trypanosomiasis.

2. A. Travel to India is associated with by far the greatest number of illness episodes. For example, travellers to Thailand have about half the chance of becoming ill when compared to those visiting India. The risk of travel-related illness is quite small in South Africa and Argentina. Risks for individual diseases vary according to location, e.g. the risk of travellers' diarrhoea is nearly 600 times greater in Nepal than in Spain. Clearly the duration of travel, the precautions taken, the activities pursued, and the age and health status of the traveller influence the risk for each individual.

3. B. *Brucella melitensis* accounts for up to 90% of brucellosis cases in humans worldwide. It is contracted by the handling or ingestion of unpasteurized milk or cheese from goats, sheep, or camels. *B. abortus* (cow), *B. suis* (pig, reindeer, caribou, and rodent), and *B. canis* (dog) are also pathogenic. Note that unprocessed cheese is not only a source of brucellosis but also a common source of listerosis. This can cause gastroenteritis or even a serious systemic illness and is especially dangerous in pregnant women.

4. D. All five types can cause death, but *P. falciparum* accounts for the vast majority of fatalities.

5. A. Lassa fever is named after a town in Nigeria. It is caused by an arena virus and is endemic in rural West Africa. The incubation period is 7–21 days. The virus is shed in the urine and saliva of multimammate rats. Infection can occur by inhalation, ingestion, or inoculation (as in hospital settings). The source of most human cases is inhalation of the virus from grain contaminated by rodent urine. Person-to-person transmission can also occur.

Most cases are subclinical but in some people the condition can progress to a severe viral hemorrhagic fever (VHF) with widespread bleeding and renal and pulmonary failure. These complications usually occur in the second week and carry a >20% mortality. Lassa fever is the most common exotic VHF to occur in the traveller.

6. C. *P. ovale* is almost exclusive to West Africa. *P. falciparum* is widely distributed but is mainly found in sub-Saharan Africa, South-East Asia and the South Pacific. *P. malariae* is found throughout Africa. *P. vivax* also occurs in Africa but is more widespread elsewhere, e.g. South-East Asia.

It is now clear that many cases of malaria in parts of South-East Asia previously thought to be due to *P. vivax* were in fact due to *P. knowlesi*. *P. knowlesi* is endemic in most of South-East Asia, including the forested areas of southern Thailand.

7. A. Falciparum malaria is found all year around in the Western Provinces of the Dominican Republic. It is still chloroquine sensitive there.

8. C. *P. knowlesi* is simian malaria and is predominantly confined to the long-tailed and pig-tailed macaque monkey of the Malaysian peninsula. It has now crossed species from monkey to humans, in whom it is sometimes fatal. It is histologically indistinguishable from *P. malariae* and can only be identified by sequencing in a malaria reference laboratory. So far it has responded well to chloroquin (2012) and mostly presents as a benign malaria, although occasionally it can be fulminating. Cases were first reported in humans in 1965 and now account for about 70% of cases in South-East Asia. Cases have also been reported in Europe in returned travellers. It is transmitted to humans and monkeys by *Anopheles latens* and *A. lucosphyrus*.

9. A. By far the highest incidence of typhoid fever is found in the Indian subcontinent followed by North Africa and Mexico. Paratyphoid A now rivals typhoid in frequency and is often as serious.

10. D. Fewer than a million *S. typhi* organisms can be infective if gastric acidity is reduced, e.g. post-vagotomy or if the person is on a proton pump inhibitor or an H2 blocker.

11. A. *S. typhi* will not survive heating above 57°C. Iodination and chlorination are also effective. *S. typhi* multiplies on cold meats and salads, and adequate sewage disposal per se will not eliminate it from the community when the personal hygiene of carriers is inadequate.

12. B. Transmission of *S. typhi* by flies and other arthropods that land on unprotected food, e.g. buffets in hotels, is probably the most common mode of spread of this disease to travellers. Consumption of sewage-infected water and shellfish is also common, although most travellers are well aware of this risk. Live *S. typhi* are initially spread by the faeco-oral route to food or to sewage from asymptomatic carriers or from a recently infected person. Droplet spread from an acute case is possible but very rare. *S. typhi* is a strict human pathogen. Most other salmonellae are zoonotic. Good personal hygiene is vital in eliminating this disease.

13. A. The estimated occurence of being bitten by a malaria-carrying mosquito is about once a week on the Kenyan coast. It rises to once a day in many parts of rural West Africa, but the risk in cities such as Kinshasa is far less. Nairobi, at 1800 m, is generally free from malaria.

The risk of malaria depends on the exact location, time of year and personal protective measures. One estimate puts the risk from travel to West Africa at 24 cases per 1000 travellers per month and from travel to Central America at 0.1 per 1000 travellers per month.

14. D. In 2007 there were 178,000 reported cases of cholera, with 4031 deaths, but the WHO estimate that these only account for 5–10% of cases worldwide. Virtually all cases reported in developed countries are imported. It is possible that 3–4 million cases occur each year, with up to 200,000 deaths. Cases have recently been reported in travellers coming from as diverse destinations as Turkey and Bali.

15. A. Leptospira enter the body through abrasions or minute cracks in the skin or mucous membrane. Immersion in or ingestion of contaminated water on white-water rafting tours is the most common way travellers get the disease. Rats excrete vast amounts of leptospira in their urine and thus contaminate rivers and soil so domestic animals such as cats and dogs are a secondary source of infection for humans.

Most reputable hotel swimming pools are free of leptospira although it can persist in surface water for several weeks. The disease has even been acquired by licking a golfball that has landed on a wet patch of grass or drinking beer directly from long-necked beer bottles. One should distinguish between black-water and white-water rafting. Black-water rafting is where the participants float through caves on tyre inner tubes. It is especially popular in New Zealand.

16. C. Viral hepatitis (HAV, HBV, HEV, and occasionally HCV) accounts for most cases of febrile jaundice in the traveller. Malaria is the second most common cause. Other causes include leptospirosis, typhoid, typhus, mononucleosis-like infections, and, rarely, viral hemorrhagic fevers and relapsing fever. Dengue fever seldom causes jaundice.

17. A. ATBF is not uncommon in travellers to southern Africa, particularly those who go on safari. *Rickettsia africae* is responsible for most cases returning from South Africa and Zimbabwe, but *R. conorii* (Mediterranean tick-borne typhus) accounts for most cases of imported typhus from the whole continent of Africa. *R. tsutsugamushi* (scrub typhus) is transmitted by larval mites to rats and humans in South-East Asia. Common findings in all three types are a skin rash, an eschar, lymphadenitis, myalgia, fever, and headache.

18. C. HAT, or sleeping sickness, is a real danger in parts of East and Central Africa. It is a zoonosis caused by *Trypanosoma brucei rhodesiense* in areas north, east, and south of Lake Victoria. It is transmitted by the tsetse fly (glossina), which bites mainly by day. The bite may be painful and the fly can even bite through thin clothing. The tsetse fly is said to be attracted to moving vehicles. A painful rubbery nodule >2.5 cm wide occurs at the site of the bite and may ulcerate to form a chancre. Adenitis and fever accompany this. All symptoms subside in a few weeks after which involvement of the central nervous system (CNS) and other organs may appear. The maximum incubation period for the initial disease is 3 weeks. *T. brucei gambiense*, which is better adapted to the human host, causes a similar disease in Western and Central Africa, often presenting later in a chronic form. HAT is endemic in 36 countries in sub-Saharan Africa. Travellers to the Serengeti are at particular risk. Pulmonary histoplasmosis is associated with exploring bat-infested caves. The traveller should receive yellow fever vaccine and advice about malaria, including chemoprophylaxis and personal protective measures against anopheles in darker hours.

19. D. The reduviid (assassin) bug that carries Chagas disease (*T. cruzi*) bites in dark shady places and mainly at night. Aedes mosquitoes, which transmit yellow fever, dengue fever and chikungunya, are daytime biters. The tsetse fly (glossina) transmits African trypanosomiasis (*T. rhodesiense* and *T. gambiense*) and bites mainly during the day. The culex mosquito, which transmits West Nile fever and Japanese encephalitis, often bites at dusk and dawn while the anopheles, which carries malaria, usually bite in darker hours. Both culex and anopheles transmit filariasis.

20. Answers: A-2; B-2; C-1; D-5; E-2; F-6

21. Answers: A-4; B-3; C-2; D-1

22. A. Viral or bacterial pharyngitis—notably 'strep throat'—is a worldwide phenomenon. Nonetheless, it is true that a sore throat is also associated with special conditions in some regions, e.g. diphtheria in Eastern Europe and the former USSR, Lassa fever in West Africa, Marburg virus, and HIV worldwide.

23. C. Protozoal cysts (giardia, cryptosporidia, cyclospora, and isospora) are only destroyed by high doses of chlorine and longer contact time than is usual in recreational swimming pools. Some parasitic eggs, e.g. ascaris, are also resistant. Enteric viruses and non-spore-forming vegetative bacteria are much more sensitive. UV treatment plant are successful in eliminating most protozoal cysts, even giardia.

24. Answers: A-2,3; B-4; C-1; D-3

25. Answers: A-3; B-4; C-2; D-5

26. Answers: A-4; B-3; C-2; D-2

27. C. Yearly death rates from wild animal attacks are not known accurately so the following figures are approximate: 65,000 for snakes, 600–800 for crocodiles, 800 for tigers and lions, 300 for elephants, 130 for hippopotamuses, 40 for hyenas, and 10–20 apiece for sharks and alligators.

28. B. The Asian black bear attacks humans in Nepal, Kashmir, India, and occasionally in Japan. Fatalities are regularly reported in the local press. Fatalities are also reported from attacks by brown bears in Siberia and the former USSR, while in India, Burma (Myanmar) and the Terrai of Nepal the sloth bear is more feared than the tiger. There are no wild bears in Africa, Australia, or New Zealand. In South America the spectacled bear is a shy forest animal that is an almost exclusive vegetarian. Deaths from attacks by grizzly and polar bears in North America are usually highlighted in the media. Fatalities from bear attacks in the USA have averaged between two and three annually since 1980.

29. C. Dengue fever is predominantly, although not exclusively, an urban disease. It is currently spreading from tropical to subtropical regions and huge numbers of people, including travellers, are contracting the disease. One is now as likely to catch dengue fever as hepatitis A when visiting South-East Asia. Chagas disease (American trypanosomiasis) is transmitted by the reduviid (triatomine) bug, bartonella (Carrion's disease) by a sandfly, and Japanese encephalitis by a culex mosquito. All three are typically rural diseases.

30. Answers: A-4; B-1; C-2; D-3

Values as reported for 2011. There are approximately 468,000 intentional homicides per year.

31. B. Currently only cholera, plague, and yellow fever are notifable to WHO.

32. A. Crude rates involve the total population of an area. Crude rates from different populations cannot be easily compared because of differences in the age and gender structure of the samples. For example, crude mortality rates in equal-number groups are higher in those locations where there are many old or sick people.

33. D. The infant mortality is the total number of deaths in the first year of life. The infant mortality rate is calculated by dividing the number of children dying under one year of age by the number of live births that year. In most countries the infant mortality rate is below 20 per 1000 live births. In upper socioeconomic groups it is less than 10 per1000 live births. In poor countries this rate may be as high as 350 per 1000 live births.

The neonatal mortality rate is the number of deaths in the first 28 days of life divided by the number of live births per year. The perinatal mortality rate is the number of stillbirths and other deaths that occur in the first 7 days of life divided by the total number of births in a year.

34. D. All statements are true. **Incidence** refers to the number of people who started a disease in a specific period. **Prevalence** refers to the number of people who are currently sick at a particular time while the **attack rate** refers to the number of people studied from a particular date and who now present with the disease.

35. B. Doxycycline is cheap and effective against many diseases besides malaria. The BCR ratio is very difficult to assess as it involves the expected prevalence of the disease, the cost of the medicine, the cost of hospitalization, the frequency, timing, and duration of travel, and the age and general condition of the traveller.

36. D. Hepatitis A vaccine gives excellent protection against the most likely disease the 'average' traveller may contract. It is effective, has few adverse side effects, and is inexpensive. The BCR of any vaccine depends on the traveller's specific itinerary, duration of stay, and risks taken.

37. B. There is a relationship between the number of new cases that arise and the duration of each case. Clearly the prevalence will rise if the incidence rises, even if the duration remains the same. Similarly the prevalence will rise if the incidence remains the same but the duration of the disease increases.

38. C. Although the number of cases of imported malaria is declining almost 10,000 cases were notified in Europe in 2010. This is probably a gross underestimate. The highest rates occur in France (8000) followed by the UK (2069), the USA (1402), Italy (986), and Germany (732). Dengue fever imports are now increasing rapidly. This is generally a mild condition, although it can be deadly in a minority of cases.

39. C. Imported malaria accounts for >80 deaths annually in Europe and about 25 deaths annually in the USA. Virtually all deaths are due to *P. falciparum* infection. The case fatality rate per 1000 is France 4, Italy 6.5, UK 8.5, USA 13, and Germany 30.4. The danger is greatest in the elderly, non-natives, VFRs and those who took incorrect or no chemoprophylaxis. Many cases originate in East Africa probably because of the great number of travellers visiting that region, which has increased since President Obama, with his Kenyan ancestry, has taken up office.

40. B. The risk of being bitten by a mosquito carrying *P. falciparum* is greatest in West Africa and some authorities put this as high as once a day in rural settings. East Africa carries the second highest risk. *P. falciparum* also occurs in Assam, the Thai–Myanmar border area, and Cambodia, in descending frequency.

41. A. Yellow fever is endemic in sub-Saharan Africa, roughly between latitudes 15°N and 20°S, and in northern parts of South America (Honduras to Bolivia, including the western two-thirds of Brazil, Venezuela, Colombia, and those parts of Peru and Ecuador that lie east of the Andes). Most cases of yellow fever have occurred after travel to West Africa. There is a current resurgence in yellow fever in Africa and in South America. Following an outbreak of yellow fever in northern Uganda in 2011 Zanzibar demanded proof of vaccination for anyone entering. A yellow-fever-like outbreak has also occurred recently in rural Kenya and Uganda. Check the current situation.

42. C. An *Aedes* index of <1.0 indicates that the danger of yellow fever in that area is nil or minimal. This depends on the fact that the mosquito vector for urban yellow fever is mostly *Aedes aegypti*. This is a peri-domestic mosquito that breeds in water that is trapped, for exapmple in tins, cans, and old tyres. Anti-mosquito measures have largely eliminated this in city centres but reinfestation can occur, especially in towns near forests, as experienced in Santa Cruz, Bolivia.

43. A. The CDC has sensibly eliminated any difference between yellow-fever-infected areas (risk areas) and yellow-fever-endemic zones (yellow fever known to exist) so that the term 'yellow-fever-endemic zone' now includes not only areas that report yellow fever cases but also those where a 'competent vector, non-human primates and ecological conditions for yellow fever virus transmission exist'. Argentina is included on this list. Some countries, e.g. Argentina, Brazil, Bolivia, and Kenya, are not holoendemic because only a part of the country carries the risk of yellow fever.

44. A. MVAs are by far the most common cause of fatal injury in travellers. Drowning comes second. Infections account for <2% of fatalities. Rates vary depending on travel area, how the traveller behaves, and local security issues. For example, homicide rates of up to 8% have been reported for travellers to highly violent areas.

45. C. A survey of British tourists found falls on land and in water sports to be the most common cause of non-fatal injury. It is likely that very severe injuries requiring medical evacuation are most commonly due to MVAs.

46. A. Global TB closely follows the incidence of HIV infection. Rates of >300 per 100,000 of population are recorded in Africa, 100–300 per 100,000 in Asia, and <10 per 100,000 in the USA and Australia. An estimated 9 million people contracted TB worldwide in 2010, with 1.5 deaths (CDC, accessed July 2012).

47. B. When DOTS is performed properly it is the best way to both prevent the spread and ensure the cure of TB. Unfortunately the relapse rate after DOTS can be as high as 14%. It is unlikely that TB is being diagnosed earlier nowadays despite careful monitoring of high-risk groups, e.g. intravenous drug abusers, those who are HIV positive, and high-risk travellers. Poverty has been shown to be an independent risk factor for TB. Stroptomycin is one of several drugs used. Remember that monotherapy with any drug for TB is inapropriate. Triple drug therapy is now the rule.

48. A. Wild ducks are the natural reservoir for H5N1 influenza. The danger is that H5N1 virus may mix with H3N2 (influenza A) and initiate a 'strain jump' such as occurred in the devastating 'flu pandemics in the past. For this reason it is important to administer 'flu vaccine to travellers to endemic areas where 'flu is not only seasonal but may be present all year round, e.g. southern Vietnam. Oseltamavir (Tamiflu®) 75 mg daily may act as a preventive during an epidemic of avian flu.

49. C. Lyme disease is caused by the spirochete *Borrelia burgdorferi* and is carried by ticks of the Ixodes species. It is associated with outdoor activity in temperate zones, particularly in forested regions of Europe and Asia and in the north-eastern, north-central and Pacific coastal regions of North America. Reported Lyme disease has doubled in the USA since 1991. It was first described in 1977 and is called after the town of Old Lyme in the USA. Lyme has not been reported to date from the Southern hemisphere but this situation is unlikely to last.

50. C. The OCP was started in West Africa (Volta river basin) in 1974. Control of the black fly (*Simulium damnosum*) has been achieved using temepos, which combines high effectiveness against the larvae, low toxicity for humans, and non-targeting of flora and fauna. Mass ivermectin treatment of the local population complements this. The Jimmy Carter Foundation has supported this project generously.

51. D. *O. volvulus* differs from other forms of filariasis in that it is the body's reaction to the dead microfilariae that causes the symptoms. Among these are intense itching, rashes, and eye lesions. Blindness is the most important lasting effect. Yearly ivermectin (Mectizan™) is recommended for those affected. Subcutaneous nodules, enclosed in fibrous tissue, occur over bony prominences. Nodules contain live and dead adult worms. The majority of cases occur in sub-Saharan Africa. The African disease is associated with lower limb nodules. Nodules on the head are typical of the South American disease. In other types of filariasis it is the live adult worms or live microflariae that cause symptoms.

52. A. The rapid epidemiological assessment for onchocerciasis (REAO) involves counting palpable nodules in 50 adult males and then extrapolating the results for the local community. However, diethylcarbamazine (DEC) skin patch testing is more convenient, more accurate, and does not cost much more.

53. C. Bathing in or contact with schistosomal-infected water is most common in sub-Saharan Africa, where up to one-third of school children may be affected. Schistosomiasis can also be acquired from the waters of the Mekong Delta. It rarely, if ever, occurs in the Amazonia and not at all in India.

54. Answers: A-2; B-3; C-3; D-5; E-1,2,4

    A-2. Athough *S. mansoni* is the predominant form found in Brazil it is also present in the Philippines and in many parts of Africa and South America, with pockets in the Yemen and Saudia Arabia. *S. mansoni* is the most widespread form of schistosoma worldwide.

    B-3. *S. japonicum* is confined to the Philippines, Indonesia, southern China, and the Yangtze basin.

    C-3. *S. japonicum* is predominant in southern China and the Yangtze basin.

    D-5. *S. mekongi* is found in the Mekong Delta region.

    E-1,2,4. *S. hematobium* is predominantly found in sub-Saharan Africa (85%), including Mozambique, with pockets along the Nile and in Yemen. *S. intercalatum* is found only in selected parts of west and central sub-Saharan Africa, e.g. Gabon, the Cameroons, and the Democratic Republic of the Congo. It causes rectal disease.

55. A. Six diseases contribute over 90% of total infectious disease deaths, probably in the following order: ARI, AIDS, diarrhoeal diseases, TB, malaria, and measles. The place of each disease in this list can be disputed. Malnutrition is a contributory factor to death in many cases.

56. A. Diarrhoeal diseases and ARIs are approximately equal causes of death in under-five-year-olds in developing countries. Measles, AIDS, malaria, and TB follow these two in probable order of frequency.

57. A. Over 90% of the 600,000 cases reported annually occur in India, Pakistan, Bangladesh, and Nepal, followed by the Sudan and north-eastern Brazil.

58. A. Parenteral transmission of leishmania, usually by blood transfusion, needle sharing or body piercing has been widely reported from Brazil and Spain. Congenital transmission also occurs. While most cases are asymptomatic, long-term damage has not been studied yet. Both *B. hominis* and Hepatitis A are transmitted via the faeco-oral route, while varicella (highly contagious) is spread by coughing and sneezing.

59. C. Dengue fever is spreading alarmingly in Asia and the Pacific regions. Control programmes for *Ae. aegypti* had almost eliminated dengue fever from South and Central America by 1970. Unfortunately DV-2 serovar was isolated in the Caribbean in 1953 and DV-3 in 1998, both presumably having come from South-East Asia. Since then dengue fever in South America has reached levels not seen since the 1930s. Despite the presence of *Ae. aegypti* in many places, e.g. parts of the USA, dengue fever outbreaks have not occurred there. While DV is widespread in Africa, dengue fever is very rare in indigenous people. This appears to be due to the presence of a dengue-resistant gene. The DV transmission cycle is person–mosquito–person. Aedes is a small daytime-biting mosquito that feeds almost exclusively on humans. It thrives in peridomestic locations and thus, not surprisingly, dengue fever is primarily an urban disease. It is interesting to note that DV has been transmitted acidentally from viraemic blood in a laboratory setting.

60. D. Changes in climate, habitat, and travel have resulted in an expansion of TBE in Europe. The first case reported in Norway was in 1998. Bornholm, an island in the Baltic, has reported the first new cases in 40 years. Tick infection rates vary from as low as 0.1% in parts of Europe to up to 40% in Siberia.

It is important that the travel health provider has some knowledge of medically important arthropods. While visual identification of some of the most common arthropods, e.g. *Culex pipiens*, is difficult, identification of others is easy, e.g. a resting female *Anopheles* spp. or an *Aedes albopictus* (tiger mosquito).

There is hardly a more neglected field in the undergraduate curriculum of nurses, doctors, and pharmacists than medical entomology.

Many well-qualified professional healthcare workers do not know that a spider has eight legs (class arachnida) or that an insect (class insecta) has six legs. Although it may seem that this information borders on trivia sometimes it may be extremely important.

1. **Which of the following is true of arthropods?**
   A. The vast majority of arthropods have four pairs of legs
   B. All arthropods have a two-segment body (head, thorax/abdomen)
   C. Arthropods make up approximately a tenth of all living organisms
   D. All arthropods are invertebrates

2. **Which of the following is true of mosquitoes?**
   A. Mosquitoes are found all over the world
   B. The female mosquitoe requires a human blood meal in order to produce eggs
   C. HIV neither survives nor replicates in mosquitoes
   D. The female mosquitoe always lays her eggs on the surface of water

3. **Which of the following is characteristic of a typical adult mosquito?**
   A. The average life span of the adult is 2–3 months
   B. The unassisted flight range seldom exceeds 100 m
   C. The usual speed of flight is between 5 and 10 km/h (3 and 6 mph)
   D. Both male and female mosquitoes feed on plant nectar

4. **Malaria is carried by**
   A. *Aedes albopictus* (Asian tiger mosquito)
   B. *Anopheles stephensi*
   C. *Culex fatigans*
   D. *Aedes aegypti*

5. **West Nile virus is transmitted by**
   A. Culex mosquitoes
   B. Bats
   C. Rat droppings
   D. Pet birds

6. **Anopheline mosquitoes are the major vectors of**
   A. *W. bancrofti*
   B. *Brugia timori*
   C. Schistosomiasis
   D. Dengue fever

7. **Mosquitoes of the genus Anopheles are easy to distinguish from those belonging to non-malaria-carrying genera because**
   A. They have six pairs of legs
   B. At rest they tilt their bodies head-down tail-up
   C. They have uniform dark-coloured wings
   D. The feelers (palpi) on either side of the central bundle (the proboscis) are short and can be distinctly seen by the naked eye

8. **Which of the following is a characteristic of female anopheline malaria-carrying mosquitoes?**
   A. *An. gambiae* is the predominant malaria-carrying species of anopheles in Africa
   B. They have four pairs of wings
   C. They are weak-sighted
   D. They lay their eggs in bundles of 40–400 at a time

9. **Mosquitoes are attracted to humans by**
   A. Lactic acid
   B. Dry skin
   C. Fair skin
   D. A fall in temperature at night

10. **Bright colours appear to attract**
    A. *Anopheles* (*gambiae* and *stephensi*)
    B. *Culex pipiens*
    C. *Glossina* (tsetse fly)
    D. *Aedes albopictus*

11. **Which of the following are effective arthropod larva control methods?**
   A. Larvivorous fish are useful when trying to clear a large area
   B. Spraying mineral oils on breeding sites should be repeated at 3-monthly intervals to be effective
   C. Of the insecticides in common use only organochlorines, e.g. DDT, have been proved useful
   D. Tipping polystyrene beads into latrines and soakaway pits can greatly inhibit larva development

12. **Which of the following is true of the common house fly, *M. domestica*?**
   A. *M. domestica* may carry methicillin-resistant *S. aureus* (MRSA) to humans
   B. *M. domestica* is a strict vegetarian
   C. *M. domestica* prefers sunlight to shade
   D. *M. domestica* commonly rests on or near the eyes

13. **Which of the following is true of black flies (Simuliidae)?**
   A. They are large flies, at least twice as long as *M. domestica*
   B. They bite at night
   C. Only females take blood meals
   D. They rarely travel more than 50 m from where they were hatched

14. **Which of the following is true of bed bugs (Cimicidae)?**
   A. They can fly up to 50 m
   B. They may carry the hepatitis B virus
   C. Only the females take a blood meal
   D. Thay have been shown to transmit the norovirus to humans

15. **Tsetse-flies (Glossinidae)**
   A. Are found in most tropical countries
   B. Lay their eggs in shady locations
   C. Have a rigid proboscis that projects straight in front of the head
   D. Blood feed once a month

16. **Most anopheles mosquitoes**
   A. Prefer to breed in polluted puddles of water
   B. Lay their eggs in groups resembling 'rafts'
   C. Have eggs that can withstand desiccation for many months
   D. Have larvae that lie parallel to the water surface

17. **Most culicine mosquitoes**
   A. Prefer to breed in dirty or polluted water
   B. Have distinct floats on their eggs
   C. Are generally larger mosquitoes than anopheles
   D. Do not have a respiratory siphon when in the larval stage

18. *Aedes aegypti*
    A. Is a night-time biter
    B. Prefers to bite people on the ankles and calves
    C. Is a native South American mosquito
    D. Flys many kilometres from its breeding place

19. **Aedes mosquitoes are important in the transmission of**
    A. Urban yellow fever virus
    B. Japanese encephalitis virus
    C. St Louis encephalitis virus
    D. West Nile virus

20. *Aedes albopictus*
    A. Can only mate with its own kind
    B. Was introduced to the USA from South America
    C. Has eggs that are destroyed by very cold winters
    D. Is an aggressive daytime biter even in the sunshine

21. **Which of the following is true of ticks?**
    A. Ticks are most abundant in wooded areas
    B. Ticks need to feed on animal blood about once every 10 days
    C. Ticks are noted for jumping down on their host
    D. Ticks may transmit disease to humans because of faulty extraction from the skin

22. *Ixodes ricinus* **(hard-backed castor-bean tick)**
    A. Needs dry weather to develop from egg to adult
    B. Can quest a host at temperatures below 5°C
    C. Can detect potential hosts by their shadows
    D. Is active up to 5000 m

23. *Ixodes ricinus* **(hard-backed castor-bean tick) is found**
    A. Free-living on the ground or among vegetation
    B. On leaves and branches at least 1.5 m above ground level
    C. Deep in forested areas
    D. On the upper surfaces of leaves and grasses

24. **After a tick attaches to a human**
    A. Only female ones can pass on disease
    B. 12 hours may pass before the tick starts to feed
    C. The tick has a maximum feeding period of 1 minute
    D. It has to have a blood meal to pass on tick-borne viral or bacterial diseases

25. Removal of ticks from the skin is best achieved by

A. Gently heating the tick
B. Extracting with a sharp forceps
C. Extracting with a blunt forceps
D. Manually pulling the tick out

26. The most dangerous medical condition associated with ticks is

A. Tick-borne typhus
B. Allergic reaction
C. Tick paralysis
D. Lyme disease

27. Which of the following is true of mites?

A. Mites differ fundamentally in structure from ticks
B. Mites transmit scabies
C. Mites thrive in mattresses
D. Mites rarely cause allergic reactions

28. Human fleas (*Pulex irritans*)

A. Can jump 60 cm (24 inches) vertically
B. Tend to bite mainly on the legs
C. Can bite at all stages of development after hatching from eggs
D. Can fly short distances

29. The human flea (*Pulex irritans*)

A. Can transmit endemic typhus
B. Can transmit cat-scratch disease
C. Can transmit Oroya fever
D. Is a strict ectoparasite

30. The triatomine bug (reduviid bug, 'kissing bug') carries

A. American trypanosomiasis (Chagas disease)
B. African trypanosomiasis (sleeping sickness)
C. New World leishmaniasis
D. Old World leishmaniasis

31. Which of the following is true of human African trypanosomiasis?

A. It is more frequently reported in long-term than in short-term travellers to disease endemic countries
B. Most cases reported by disease endemic countries are due to *T. rhodesiense*
C. Anti-trypanosomal drugs are now widely available
D. A chancre at the site of the tsetse fly bite is typical of most *T. rhodesiense* infections

1. D. The phylum Arthropoda makes up nearly 80% of all known living animals, ranging from microscopic marine species to terrestrial insects such as ticks, mites, fleas, and mosquitoes. Size varies from very small, e.g. some microscopic marine species, to very large, e.g. the king crab with its span of around 3.2 m (12 feet).

All known arthropods are cold-blooded invertebrates with segmented bodies encased in a hard chitinous exoskeleton. The name arthropod is derived from their characteristic jointed appendages. One or two pairs of appendages are linked to each body segment and so their number depends on the number of segments present. Consequently, leg numbers vary from three pairs, e.g. butterflies, beetles, and ants, to four pairs in the arachnid class to 18 or more pairs in centipedes and millipedes. It is debated whether or not all arthropods evolved from one or more distinct arthropod ancestor (velvet worms, onychophora).

2. C. HIV neither survives nor replicates in the mosquito and thus mosquitoes do not spread HIV. Only female anthropophilic mosquitoes require a human blood meal in order to produce eggs. The vast majority are zoonophilic and only use animal blood. Although eggs are usually laid on the surface of water or on land that is likely to be flooded, some eggs may survive months in a desiccated state until the environment is right for hatching.

Mosquitoes are found everywhere except in the Antarctic. The Arctic teems with mosquitoes in the summer time. *Ochlerotatus communis*, which occurs north of the Arctic circle, is such an aggressive biter that it will feed on the blood of dead caribou.

3. D. Both sexes live on plant nectar, but females must also have blood protein (human or animal depending on species) in order to produce eggs. Less than 10% of female *An. gambiae* survive longer than 2 weeks but many other mosquitoes can live up to 3 weeks but not 2–3 months. No mosquito can keep up with someone walking briskly since they only fly at up to 1–2 km/h (1.0–1.5 mph). Unassisted, some can fly several kilometres and remain airborne for 4–5 hours. High winds can blow mosquitoes long distances. Note that *Ae. albopictus* has a short flight range and, like the more common *Ae. aegypti*, is a peridomestic mosquito, that is, it likes to live near human habitations. Note that although *Ae. aegypti* is a daytime biter it also bites at night where there is artificial lighting. It is best known as the carrier of the yellow fever and dengue viruses. The brightly coloured Asian tiger mosquito (*Ae. albopictus*) is an aggressive biter, but although it transmits dengue in the tropics, it does not seem to have done so in the southern USA despite a rapid increase in its numbers there. *Ae. albopictus* actively seeks out its human and animal prey.

4. B. All these mosquitoes bite humans and all may carry disease. The subfamily anopheles is the one responsible for transmitting malaria. Nonetheless, of the many different species of anopheles, only about 484 are of medical importance and different species carry malaria in different parts of the world. For example, *An. stephensi* is a major malaria vector in the cities and coastal regions of India and Pakistan, while *An. gambiae* is probably the major malaria vector in Africa.

Although culicine mosquitoes are often regarded as merely a nuisance they too can transmit disease, e.g. filariasis.

5. A. West Nile virus is transmitted by ornithophilic culex species, especially by *Cx. quinquefasciatus* ('quinks') and to a lesser extent by *Anophele* spp. 'Quinks' are also the chief vector of St Louis encephalitis, western equine encephalitis and of Bancroftian filariasis (especially in cities). *Cx. tritaeniorhynchus* transmits Japanese encephalitis. *Cx. tritaeniorhynchus* can fly up to 4.82 km (3 miles) on its own and over 48.2 km (30 miles) on a favourable wind. It is not known whether or not chemical repellents are effective against *Cx. tritaeniorhynchus*.

Culex is a night-time biter and is the main mosquito to cause the well-known 'buzzing' sound, caused by beating its wings (250–500 times per second). The buzz is common to both males and females, and is probably used as a sexual signal between them.

6. A. Apart from malaria, anopheles transmit lymphatic filariasis (*W. bancrofti*) and some arboviruses. e.g. o'nyong-nyong. Culex and anopheles carry lymphatic filariasis, but the mansonia mosquito is the major vector of *B. timori filariasis*. Schistosomiasis is transmitted from fresh water snails by infective cerceriae. Dengue fever is chiefly transmitted by *Ae. aegypti*.

7. B. 'Bottom up' is the typical resting stance of anopheles. Other mosquitoes hold themselves more or less parallel to the surface when they rest. Like many mosquitoes anopheles have three pairs of jointed legs and most have distinctive dappled wings, giving the appearance of alternating blocks of light and shade. Unlike other mosquitoes it is difficult to see the palpi as discreet entities.

8. A. *An. gambiae* is the major malaria-carrying mosquito in Africa. Recently its genome has been encoded, raising hopes of intervention at the vector stage of this disease. *An. gambiae* mosquitoes are attracted to humans by smell and movement. They have two compound eyes with good vision that also aids in locating their victim. Unlike their culex cousins, anopheline mosquitoes lay 30–150 eggs singly, every 2–3 days. All mosquitoes, and all true flies, are Diptera and only have two wings. This distinguishes true flies from false flies, e.g. mayflies, dragonflies, butterflies, and fireflies.

9. A. Mosquitoes have chemoreceptors on their antennae that are stimulated by lactic acid. They are also attracted by wet or sweaty skin, warm skin, CO_2, perfumes, and apocrine and eccrine secretions. The fall in ambient temperature at night appears to have little effect.

10. C. Glossina are attracted to bright (especially blue) or contrasting colours and to the dust and motion of vehicles. They can also bite through clothing. Avoiding tsetse-fly bites is thus almost impossible for anyone visiting an endemic area over a long period. Furthermore, there is little evidence that proprietary insect repellents prevent glossina biting, although glossina can be killed by knock-down repellents such as permethrin. Anopheles and culex are attracted to darker colours but information about aedes and colour attraction is sketchy.

11. D. Larvivorous fish such as gambusia, carp, guppy, and tilapia are difficult to control, unpredictable in behaviour, and only useful in limited locations. There are numerous larvicidal bacteria and viruses available and of these *Bacillus thuringiensis* Israeli (BTI) is the most widely used. It is non-toxic to humans and wildlife, easily mass-produced and available in long-acting forms.

Spraying with mineral oil must be repeated once a week in the tropics. It is expensive and very much hit and miss.

Chemical control involves expense, uncertain environmental effects, and the danger of entry of the substance into the human food chain, as with DDT. Nonetheless DDT is a really powerful insecticide and is coming back into favour.

Cx. quinquefasciatus is a vector for filariasis, West Nile fever and St Louis encephalitis. It preferentially breeds in polluted waters such as pit latrines and clogged drains. Tipping in polystyrene beads to form a floating layer 1–2 cm thick can prevent breeding, thereby suffocating the larvae. This has been done to good effect in parts of India and Zanzibar.

12. A. In 2004 a report from the city hospital in Misurata, Libya showed the transfer of MRSA by houseflies. *M. domestica* transmits pathogens (viruses, bacteria, spirochetes, and protozoans) by defaecation, contaminated feet and mouthparts (especially shigella), and vomiting on food during feeding, a common occurrence. The housefly eats anything from rotting meat to vegetables to milk. It prefers shade to sunlight, and rarely rests near the eyes except for some varieties, such as the latrine fly. This is found mainly in Africa and is important in transmitting trachoma.

13. C. Female black flies are the only vector of human onchocerciasis (river-blindness). Their mouthparts are ideally suited for introducing infective larvae and at the same time sucking up any microfilariae that are already in the skin. They bite only during the day, especially during the early morning and late afternoon. Although they are only 1.4–4 mm long they can travel long distances (2–100 km) even without the aid of the wind. The eggs of *S. damnosum*, which is the main black fly vector of onchocerciasis, are laid in favoured sites near the banks of rivers or on submerged vegetation or on stones in streams, usually fast-flowing oxygenated streams. It is useful to know that the bite of the black fly is usually painful.

14. B. Bed bugs have no wings and cannot fly. During the day bed bugs hide in dark dry places, e.g. mattresses, cracks in walls, furniture, and wallpaper. Both sexes emerge at night to feed on sleeping people and return to their hideouts to digest their blood meals. Backpackers who are familiar with numerous dark brown or black spots on bed linen in hostels may be happy to know that these are the excreta of bed bugs and are not in themselves going to affect them. Although hepatitis B virus and at least 27 other pathogens have been found in bed bugs, they do not seem to pass disease on to people, and the bugs themselves are to be avoided mainly for their intense nuisance value. Their presence also indicates a poor level of housing and cleanliness.

15. C. The rigid straight proboscis, the closed cell between wing veins that resembles a hatchet, wings folded scissor-like over the body, and a size of 8–12 mm all make identification of tsetse flies easy. These flies are unusual in that they lay larvae not eggs and in that both males and females take blood feeds every 2–3 days, despite resting for 23 of the 24 hours.

Both sexes are vectors of trypanosomiasis. Feeding on any handy animal (humans, beasts, birds) occurs during the daytime. Tsetse flies are limited to sub-Saharan Africa apart from two species found in south-west Arabia.

16. D. Anopheles larvae, unlike culicines, lie parallel just under the water surface. This is useful as they are surface feeders and mostly develop in water not polluted by organic material. They lay their eggs singly and have a distinctive pair of lateral air-filled sacs, called 'floats'. Anopheles eggs hatch in 2–3 days in warm climates but cannot withstand desiccation at any temperature.

17. A. The important medical culicine genera are Aedes, Culex, Mansonia, Haemagogus, Sabethes, and Psorophora. Although one medically important species, *Cx. quinquefasciatus* (vector of bancroftian filariasis), breeds in polluted water, other types of culicine mosquito, e.g. Aedes, prefer clean water and some, e.g. *Ae. albopictus* (the tiger mosquito), prefer to breed in sheltered water holes, e.g. rot holes in trees, coconut husks, old tyres, and bamboo stumps.

Culicine eggs never have floats but all culicine larvae possess respiratory siphons and so lie at an angle below the water surface, in contrast to anopheles. Culicines are mostly the same size as anopheles (5–7 mm) although a few genera are smaller, e.g. *C. sonorensis* (2 mm). Note that the names *Stegomyia aegypti* and *S. albopictus* have been correctly assigned to what were formerly known as *Ae. aegypti* and *Ae. albopictus*. However, many of us still continue to use the older more familiar taxonomy.

18. B. *Ae. aegypti* typically bites on the ankles and this explains why many people in endemic areas constantly twitch their legs to frighten them off. Aedes are very sensitive to movement and flirt away if you twitch, only to land and bite elsewhere. This is sometimes called the 'babu bounce' and is widespread in India. It is recognized by the constant twitching of legs seen sometimes when a group of people are sitting in an office or waiting room. Aedes originated in Africa and was probably carried via slave ships to the Bahamas in the 1600s. *Ae. aegypti* breeds in dark places near human habitation and can only fly a few hundred metres. It is a daytime biter but will bite at night in illuminated areas, e.g. in houses and garage forecourts. It appears to have a preference for human blood over animal blood.

19. A. *Ae. aegypti* and *Ae. albopictus* are both involved in the urban yellow fever virus cycle where human-to-human transmission occurs. Sylvatic yellow fever virus transmission occurs via *Ae. africanus* in Africa and *Haemagogus spegazzini* in South and Central America.

As noted above, culex mosquitoes are primarily responsible for transmitting Japanese encephalitis virus, St Louis encephalitis virus, and West Nile virus. In contrast to *Ae. aegypti* and *Ae. albopictus* culex bite throughout the night, although they are most active towards sundown (crepuscular) and up to 1 hour after sunrise.

20. D. *Ae. albopictus* is also called the Asian tiger mosquito because of its black and white body stripes and the distinctive single white stripe down its back. It will leave its shady resting place and bite even in the noonday sun. Unlike *Ae. aegypti* it is very resistant to cold and the male can mate with other species of mosquitoes. This can render the latter sterile so the local mosquito population can be wiped out in a short time.

Both *Ae. aegypti* and *Ae. albopictus* are categorized as peridomestic, diurnally active, tree-hole breeding mosquitoes.

Ae. albopictus is believed to have been imported into the USA and other countries, e.g. Canada, Brazil, and Australia, in the late 1970s in motor tyres that which were due for re-threading. The imported tyres came mainly from Japan and Taiwan, where this process was illegal.

Ae. albopictus is a 'container' breeder, that is, it thrives in puddles that gather in old tyres, discarded coke tins, buckets, and gutters. It can carry many viruses, e.g. DV, la Crosse encephalitis, and West Nile virus, and has the potential to act as a link between sylvatic and urban yellow fever. *Ae. albopictus* has spread worldwide and is now found in many places, e.g. the Dominican Republic, Nigeria, Albania, the Netherlands, France, Belgium, Spain, and in particular in northern Italy.

21. D. Improper removal of ticks, in which the stomach contents are squeezed, can readily transmit disease, e.g. erlichiosis and tick-borne encephalitis. In general, ticks are found in tall grass and shrubbery, not often in woods. They never jump down, they always move against gravity. Ticks feed only once on animal blood at each stage of development (larva, nymph, adult) and can go for years without a feed.

22. C. Haller's organ, on the tick's forelegs, detects the shadow, body heat, odours, and vibrations of a prospective host. Ticks only thrive in high humidity (>85%) and quest hosts only in environments >7°C. Ticks are small arachnids and not insects. Both insects and ticks are arthropods. Tick saliva concentrates pathogens such as tick borne encephalitis virus, *Borrelia burgdorferi* (Lyme disease), *Babesia microti* (babesiosis), and many other bacteria, parasites, and toxins. Global warming has allowed ticks to thrive at altitudes >1000 m and even through the winter in many sheltered parts of Europe. Adult females and nymphs can transmit infections through their bites. Male ticks attach to but do not feed for long on humans. Female ticks may increase their body size 200-fold during a blood meal.

23. A. The common hard-backed castor-bean tick (*Ixodes ricinus*) spends most of its life on the underside of leaves, grasses, and foliage less than 1.5 m high. It prefers to face a sunny aspect and groups of ticks tend to accumulate towards the tips of vegetation, where they drop off or are brushed off by animals and humans. Riverbanks and grassy meadows, especially where benches and barbecue facilities are provided, provide an excellent habitat for ticks.

24. B. Both male and female ticks pass on disease by injecting infected saliva into an appropriate host. Over 95% of ixodes are three-host ticks, that is they bite a different host, not necessarily a different species, at each stage of development (larva, nymph, adult). This facilitates disease spread in contrast to one-host ticks, which stay on the same host throughout their lives. Male ixodes suck out tissue fluid and bite more often than females and thus are potentially more dangerous in transmitting disease than females although they do not feed for as long a time as females. Both sexes engorge with host blood during a meal and so host disease, e.g. viral encephalitis, is transferred to the tick in this way. After attachment it may take 12–24 hours before feeding begins. Only about 1% of tick bites cause disease. Ticks feed for a maximum of 15 minutes.

Many ticks are very small and difficult to see, yet one bite can cause disease.

Ticks are the major cause of arthropod-borne disease after mosquitoes.

25. C. Gently extract the tick with a blunt forceps, making sure not to crush the head or leave any parts behind. Painting with petroleum, vaseline, or alcohol is useless, although spraying or painting with an insect repellent may prevent the tick from injecting its saliva and cause it to fall off naturally in 24 hours. The use of sharp forceps, manual removal, twisting, or squishing the tick is contraindicated and may cause salivation and regurgitation of tick contents into the damaged skin.

26. B. Allergic reactions can vary from mild itching to an imminent life-threatening catastrophe. Furthermore, allergic reactions can occur when one is bitten at any stage of a tick's development. Anyone who has had even a minor reaction in the past must totally avoid contact with tick-infested areas.

Tick paralysis, most often seen in children, is caused by a bite from the 'paralysis tick', *Ixodes holocyclus*. This is the most medically important tick in eastern Australia. The development of an antitoxin has prevented deaths from this condition for the past 70 years.

Lyme disease and tick typhus are readily cured by tetracyclines if given early enough.

27. C. Mites thrive in warm humid places such as mattresses, upholstery, tapestries, carpets, draperies, stuffed toys, and clothes. Both mites and ticks belong to the same family, Acari, and are both arthropods. Dust mites are second only to pollen in causing allergic reactions. Mites do not carry scabies, they are scabies; *Sarcoptes scabiei* is a mite.

S. scabiei burrow into the skin and cause severe itching (scabere, to itch), which is worst at night. Humanitarian workers in close contact with local populations and tourists staying in cheap accommodation should beware of contact with mites. The dust mite thrives on human skin scales while others actually bite humans (tropical rat mite) and cause dermatitis and blistering of the skin. Mites are generally too small to be seen by the naked eye. Mites create many problems for domestic and wild animals.

28. B. Fleas are wingless biting insects that are common pests of domestic dogs and cats as well as other animals. They can jump vertically up to 18 cm (7 inches) and horizontally up to 33 cm (13 inches). Fleas from dogs, cats, rats, and mice occasionally spread diseases such as plague, typhus, and even tapeworms. They are annoying to both people and pets, and commonly cause skin irritation with itching and infection. They have four stages of development (ova, larva, pupa, adult) but only adult fleas (5% of the flea population) bite humans.

The Black Death or bubonic plague (1347–1350) was caused by infection with *Pasteurella (yersinia) pestis* injected with the saliva of the oriental rat flea (*Xenopsylla cheopsis*). Nowadays the danger is remote although still extant in Vietnam, India, and some parts of South America and Africa. Plague vaccine is rarely used.

29. D. The human flea is a strict ectoparasite and does not invade beneath the skin. Human fleas will not infect humans with any disease, unlike rat, cat, and dog fleas, which carry disease from the host to humans. The human flea also infests cats, dogs, and in particular pigs. Pigsties abound with them.

Endemic typhus (*Rickettsia typhi* or *R. felis*) is spread to humans by the bite of an infected rat flea or by rubbing its faeces into a small cut or abrasion. Cat fleas cause endemic typhus (*R. felis*) in the same way. Catscratch fever (*Bartonella henselae*) is mostly caused by bites from infected domestic cats, especially kittens. Oroya fever (*B. bacilliformis*) is endemic in the Andes and is transmitted by sandflies.

30. A. *Trypanozoma cruzi* (South America) and *T. sanguisuga* (North America) are carried by triatomine infestans or the 'kissing bug'. This name is given because of its propensity to bite humans in the perioral or periorbital regions. Triatomines nest in roofs, ceilings, and wall cracks. At night they glide down on sleeping humans directed by heat sensors in their antennae. They can drift over 100 m in favourable air currents and this enables them to colonize whole villages. There is a large reservoir of trypanosomes in warm-blooded animals such as rodents. Human African trypanosomiasis is transmitted by *Glossina* spp. (tsetse fly), which is found only in rural Africa. The West African disease is caused by *T. brucei gambienes* and the East African disease by *T. brucei rhodesiense*. All pathogenic leishmania are carried by the sandfly.

31. D. The vast majority of cases in travellers are due to *T. rhodesiense*, but the majority of cases reported from endemic countries are due to *T. gambiense*. This appears to reflect the country where exposure takes place.

In one study more than 75% of HAT cases due to *T. rhodesiense* presented with a chancre. This, combined with a short exposure-symptom time (1–3 weeks post exposure) and a high parasitaemia, facilitates the diagnosis in travellers. Gambiense infections are diagnosed later (3–12 months, WHO) and are often confused with other conditions. In both infections there may be enlarged neck glands, sub-acute fever, headache, and behavioural changes. Cerebral spinal fluid (CSF) examination is helpful in such cases. Apart from pentamidine, only WHO distributes anti-HAT drugs (suramin, melarsoprol, and eflornithine).

Helminthiasis is rampant in poorer tropical countries, in fact one is surprised if a patient's stool is clear of ova or parasites when working in such places. Travellers are also liable to acquire helminthiasis from contaminated food or water, as well as via the faeco-oral route. In the latter case it may be unfair to blame poor personal hygiene since washing and sanitation facilities are often below standard. Nonetheless, the helminth load in travellers is considerably less than that in indigenous people, so the ultimate ill-effects are usually less marked in the visitor.

1. Which is the most common gut helminth found in the traveller?

   A. *Ascaris lumbricoides*

   B. *Enterobius vermicularis*

   C. *Taenia saginata*

   D. *Trichuris trichiura*

2. Which gut helminth is *most likely* to cause diarrhoea?

   A. *Ascaris lumbricoides* (common 'roundworm')

   B. *Enterobius vermicularis* (threadworm)

   C. *Trichuris trichiura* (whipworm)

   D. *Taenia species* (tapeworm)

3. The anti-helminthic mebendazole is useful in

   A. *Trichuris trichiura*

   B. *Strongyloides stercoralis*

   C. *Taeniasis* (tapeworm)

   D. *Cutaneous larva migrans* (CLM)

4. Which of these is most likely to infect pork in South-East Asia?

   A. *Taenia asiatica*

   B. *Taenia solium*

   C. *Taenia saginata*

   D. *Gnathosoma* spp. (*G. spinigerum, G. hispidum*)

5. *Strongyloides stercoralis*

A. Is confined to tropical and subtropical climates

B. Exhibits the property of 'autoinfection' in humans

C. Has been know to grow to 6 m in length

D. Is sometimes transmitted by a mosquito

6. Acute strongyloidosis (AS)

A. Is a hyperinfection syndrome

B. Is easily confused with acute schistosomiasis (Katayama syndrome)

C. Is one of the most common enteric parasites in travellers

D. Is best treated by thiabendazole

7. Cysticercosis

A. Generally becomes symptomless when the parasite dies

B. Normally has cysts <15 cm in diameter

C. Is only satisfactorily diagnosed when the larvae of *T. solium* are identified in the stool

D. Only occurs in humans

8. Neurocysticercosis (NCC)

A. Refers to infection of the CNS due to the adult stages of *Taenia solium*

B. Is caused by eating *Taenia solium*-infected raw or undercooked pork

C. Is the most common cause of acquired epilepsy in developing countries

D. Generally manifests itself symptomatically within 6 months of its acquisition

9. The primary treatment for seizures due to NCC is

A. Surgical excision of offending cyst(s)

B. Prompt administration of ivermectin

C. Prompt administration of praziquantel (PZQ)

D. Prompt administration of anti-epileptics

10. Hydatid disease

A. Has a worldwide distribution

B. Occurs chiefly in the lungs

C. Represents the adult form of the dog tapeworm (*Echinococcus* spp.)

D. Is usually associated with a marked eosinophilia

1. B. *E. vermicularis* (pinworm) is very common even in the developed world. It is spread by the faeco-oral route and both finger sucking and nail biting have also been implicated. Eggs can be inhaled as an aerosol when shaking out contaminated linen or clothes. It is said to be present in excess of 60% of children in India. The typical symptom of intense anal pruritus, especially in the evening, is due to the migration of gravid females intent on expelling their eggs in the perineum and perianal regions. Albendazole or mebendazole kills the adults—not the eggs—so that treatment should be repeated in 2 weeks in order to eliminate new adults. Personal hygiene and washing of clothes and bed linen is essential to finally eliminate the condition.

2. C. Any of the worms listed can be associated with diarrhoea, but *T. trichiura* is the most likely one. Light infestations are asymptomatic but heavier ones cause symptoms similar to inflammatory bowel disease. The adults embed in the mucosa of the caecum, colon, and rectum, and heavy infestation may result in rectal prolapse in children. Infection occurs when eggs are swallowed so that faeco-oral spread is rampant in many parts of the world.

3. A. Mebendazole (100 mg bid × 3 days), repeated if necessary, is a time-honoured antihelminthic used world wide against Trichuris, Ascaris, Enterobius, and selected hookworm infections but is ineffective against Strongyloides, Taeniasis, and Cutaneous larva migrans. Like other benzimidazoles it is potentiated by cimetidine and by steroids. In general it is less effective than albendazole apart from treatment of trichuris, where it is superior. Ivermectin is recommended against *S. stercoralis* and CLM, and niclosamide is recommended against tapeworm.

4. A. Asian pork tapeworm (*T. asiatica*) is common in South-East Asia. It is morphologically similar to *T. saginata* (beef tapeworm) and is far less likely to cause cysticercosis than *T. solium*, the traditional pork tapeworm. Gnathosoma is found in undercooked or raw fish, chicken, frogs, and reptiles.

5. B. Strongyloides is a world-wide soil-transmitted helminth mainly found in the warm moist soil of the tropics. It is never transmitted by a mosquito.

Slender 2-mm long female adults live in the mucosa of the small intestine of humans. They release eggs that rapidly turn into rhabditiform (R-form) larvae, which are excreted with the faeces. A unique free-living stage now occurs, in which infective filariform (F-form) larvae are produced. These can die, pierce intact human skin directly, or enter via contaminated food, where human faeces is used as a fertilizer ('night soil'). Another option is 'autoinfection'. In this the R-form larva changes directly into the infective F-form in the human intestine and thus re-infects by directly penetrating the intestinal mucosa.

6. B. Fever, cough, urticaria, eosinophilia, and diarrhoea may be present in Katayama fever and occasionally in other helminth infections.

The key element in Katyama fever is exposure to fresh water. The key element in acute strongyloides is walking barefoot or eating suspect food in endemic regions. Two cases were acquired in Koh Samui (Thailand) in 2008. However, in general, acute strongyloidosis is rare in travellers. Chronic or well-established strongyloidosis can present as classical evanescent larva currens due to tissue larval migration under the skin. Life-threatening hyperinfection is liable to occur years after the primary infection should the patient become immunocompromised (HIV, steroids, irradiation, chemotherapy, leukaemia, lymphoma). Ivermectin 200 µg/kg/day × 3 days or albendazole 400 mg bid × 7 days is probably the best treatment. Thiabendazole, although cheaper, is less effective and prone to more adverse side effects.

7. B. The human intestine is the definitive location for *T. solium*. Pigs are intermediate hosts in which cysticerci (containing larvae) are found. When humans accidentally become intermediate hosts by ingesting the eggs of *T. solium*, one or more small cysticercal nodules appear in various locations, especially in the CNS (85%), skeletal muscle, eye, and skin. These may be misdiagnosed as multiple lipomata, sebaceous cysts, myomata, or even muscle necrosis, as occurred in the case of one traveller. Microscopy of an excised 'cyst' usually shows typical larvae each with four suckers. Immunology, CT, and MRI scans are important tools. Often old cysts may be seen as small calcified bodies on plain X-ray.

Symptoms depend on size, number, location, and state of cyst activity. Symptoms become worse when the parasite breaks up and dies because the body launches an immediate and often dramatic inflammatory/allergic reaction.

8. C. NCC is due to larva-containing cysts of *T. solium*, and not the adult stage of *T. solium*, in the CNS. NCC is the most common parasitic disease of the CNS in poorer countries, where it is also the most common cause of acquired epilepsy. It may be responsible for 30–50% of seizures in South and Central America and India. A report from Israel (2011) showed that NCC is rare in Israeli travellers, with an estimate of 1:275,000 per travel episode to high-risk areas. Male sex, duration of travel, and careless personal habits facilitate infestation. Fits were the chief presenting feature.

'Measly' pork contains the larval stage of the worm so that ingestion of this can cause human taeniasis. In this the adult tapeworm develops and adheres to the mucosa of the upper third of the small intestine by specialized suckers. Adults worms often reach lengths of 5–10 m, live for 25 years, and produce 50,000 eggs a day, which are shed in the stool.

NCC takes >6 months to manifest itself clinically.

NCC is acquired by the faeco-oral route from egg-contaminated water, food, or fomites.

A nice demonstration that eating undercooked measly pork is not responsible for NCC is the fact that there was an outbreak of NCC in non-pork-eating orthodox Jews in New York.

9. D. Anti-epileptics should be the primary drugs in controlling seizures. Series from travellers show that a combination of antiepileptics and albendazole or PZQ is associated with the disappearance of symptoms and the shrinkage of cysts. This may not apply to NCC in endemic areas, where there is often a heavy parasite load and multiple cysts. Surgical excision is considered unnecessary and dangerous. Ivermectin is used for a wide variety of helminths, e.g. filariasis and even selected mites, e.g. sarcoptes scabei.

10. A. Hydatid disease occurs worldwide. It is due to the ingestion by humans or herbivores, especially sheep, of the ova of the dog tapeworm. The eggs reach the human liver (70%), lungs (20%), or elsewhere (10%), where they develop into classical hydatid cysts. Symptoms only occur when a cyst enlarges and presses on important structures or the cyst ruptures, resulting in an acute allergic reaction (eosinophilia at this stage) or cysts become secondarily infected.

Rupture of a pulmonary cyst will produce salty clear sputum or may result in a pneumothorax or empyema. Eating raw carcasses riddled with cysts infects dogs and related canines.

Turkana has the highest prevalence of hydatid disease in the world because of the intimate contact there between man and dog. Treatment is with albendazole or mebendazole and most cysts can be aspirated rather than excised surgically.

VACCINES

A working knowledge of vaccinology is essential for anyone involved in travel medicine. This includes the storage, indications, scheduling, common side effects, usefulness, technique of administration and management of acute adverse reactions to any vaccine one gives.

Those who administer vaccines should also be fully aware of the type of vaccine they are giving, should know exactly what is in the vaccine in question, should know its expected efficacy, and be able to roughly estimate a BCR. Giving unnecessary vaccines is reprehensible and unworthy of any doctor or nurse.

In travel medicine, the 'patient', who is normally a healthy person, must be informed of the pros and cons of any proposed vaccine. Giving vaccines is only a part of the pre-travel consultation and is certainly not the most important part.

General vaccinology

1. **Which of the following is true for vaccine administration?**
    A. Subcutaneous (SC) injections are more quickly absorbed than intramuscular (IM) ones
    B. A standard BD micro lance™ 26G (0.45 × 10 mm) needle is adequate for routine IM administration of vaccines to adults
    C. Skeletal muscle has a richer supply of pain fibres than SC tissue
    D. Skeletal muscle is more vascular than SC tissue

2. **The IM route is preferred to the SC one**
    A. When the patient has a bleeding tendency
    B. When giving live viral vaccines
    C. When giving potentially irritating vaccines
    D. When avoiding too rapid dissemination of a vaccine

3. **Which of the four choices below involve active immunization?**
    A. Tetanus immune globulin
    B. Hyperimmune rabies serum
    C. Genetically engineered vaccines such as DNA and RNA vaccines
    D. Live vaccines only when given by the parenteral route

4. **Live vaccines**

   A. Have poor efficacy if given orally
   B. Generally require a repeat dose within 6 weeks to induce satisfactory protection
   C. Evoke excellent B-cell but little or no T-cell response
   D. May cause the disease in the recipient

5. **Killed (inactivated) vaccines**

   A. May replicate within an immunodeficient recipient
   B. Require multidose immunization schedules
   C. Stimulate cellular rather than humoral immunity
   D. Are free from adjuvants

6. **Conjugate vaccines**

   A. Are created by attaching a weak antigen to a carrier protein
   B. Are especially useful in protecting older people
   C. Are most often used to create vaccines against viral infections
   D. Generally convert T-cell dependent antigens into T-cell independent ones

7. **As a general rule when giving a conjugate vaccine**

   A. It is safe to give it at the same time as a non-conjugate vaccine
   B. Allow at least a 4-week interval before giving a polysaccharide vaccine
   C. Let it precede a polysaccharide vaccine (no time limit)
   D. Be sure to allow 2 weeks to elapse before and after giving a non-conjugate polysaccharide vaccine

8. **Which of the following is true for polysaccharide vaccines?**

   A. It is not necessary to keep them in a fridge
   B. Only capsular polysaccharide vaccines should be given to children <2 years old
   C. Coupling with a protein carrier renders the polysaccharide antigen visible to T cells
   D. Booster shots are necessary

9. **It is necessary to restart an interrupted series in the case of which of the following?**

   A. Oral typhoid vaccine
   B. Rabies
   C. Hepatitis B
   D. Primary polio series with oral polio vaccine (OPV)

10. **If a subject is certain that he or she is hypersensitive to 'antibiotics' you should take special care in giving**

    A. Yellow fever vaccine
    B. Japanese encephalitis vaccine (Ixiaro™)
    C. MMR
    D. Parenteral polio vaccine

11. **Which of the following vaccines contains egg protein?**
    A. Measles
    B. Rubella
    C. Hepatitis A
    D. Hepatitis B

12. **A patient develops pruritus and rash 15 minutes after receiving travel vaccinations for Peru. This is most likely to be**
    A. A mild transitory allergic reaction
    B. A severe allergic reaction
    C. Anaphylactic shock
    D. Vasovagal attack (simple faint)

13. **Which is the most important single drug to give in anaphylaxis?**
    A. Adrenaline (epinephrine)
    B. Atropine
    C. Hydrocortisone
    D. Chlorpheniramine (antihistamine)

Specific vaccines

1. **Which of the following is true for tetanus vaccine?**
    A. It should be considered for every traveller
    B. Not more than six anti-tetanus shots should be given to anyone in their lifetime
    C. Reactions to the vaccine are less likely the greater the number of times it is given
    D. Tetanus dipsticks or automated tetanus antibody immunity testing are poorly specific for tetanus

2. **WHO states that 'vaccination against meningococcal disease is not a requirement for entry' into any countries or places or circumstance except**
    A. For pilgrims doing the Hajj
    B. Northern Nigeria during the rainy season
    C. Iran all year round
    D. Islamabad (Pakistan) during the monsoons

3. **Which of the following is true for yellow fever vaccine?**
    A. It gives < 50% protection after 10 days
    B. Protection declines fairly rapidly after 10 years
    C. It should not be given on same day as a live vaccine
    D. It is contraindicated in children < 9 months old

4. **Which of the following countries requires proof of yellow fever vaccination on entry?**

   A. Chile
   B. Madagascar
   C. Zimbabwe
   D. Angola

5. **For which one of the following countries would you recommend giving yellow fever vaccine?**

   A. Uruguay
   B. Mozambique
   C. Paraguay
   D. South Africa

6. **Which of the following is true for yellow fever vaccination?**

   A. A booster dose must be given at least 10 days before travel to an endemic area
   B. Avoid giving oral typhoid vaccine at the same visit
   C. Most vaccine-related deaths have been in children under 9 months of age
   D. A skin test should be done on anyone with a questionable history of gelatin allergy

7. **Yellow fever vaccine-associated neurotropic disease (YFVA-ND)**

   A. Is more likely after a second or subsequent dose of vaccine
   B. Is mainly confined to infants <9 months old
   C. Is equally common in the elderly as in children
   D. Has a mortality of almost 100%

8. **Yellow fever vaccine-associated viscerotropic disease (YFVA-VD)**

   A. Is most common in the elderly
   B. Is more common in females than in males
   C. Is associated with problems of the thyroid gland
   D. Only occurs in those who have had yellow fever vaccination previously

9. **Yellow fever vaccine 0.5 ml SC is contraindicated in**

   A. Elderly patients with cardiac disease
   B. Patients with a temperature >38.5°C
   C. Asymptomatic HIV+ patients with a CD4 count >400 cells/ml
   D. People with a vague history of egg allergy

10. **Yellow fever vaccine should not be given if the recipient**

    A. Is on chloroquine
    B. Is on mefloquine
    C. Takes live oral typhoid vaccine (Ty21a) at the same visit
    D. Gets BCG at the same visit

11. **Quadrivalent meningococcal capsular polysaccharide vaccine (MPSV4)**
    A. Is conjugated with protein
    B. Is given in a two-dose schedule 2–4 weeks apart
    C. Provides protection for 5–10 years in adults
    D. Is poorly immunogenic in children under 4 years of age

12. **Quadrivalent meningococcal vaccine conjugated with *Corynebacterium diphtheriae* CRM$_{197}$ protein (MCV4)**
    A. Is in the final stages of being released on the market
    B. Is primarily used for infants under 2 years of age
    C. Is recommended between 2 and 55 years of age
    D. Is less immunogenic than *ACWYvax*

13. **Which of the following is a live vaccine?**
    A. Varicella vaccine
    B. Parenteral polio vaccine
    C. Pneumoccoal vaccine
    D. Anthrax vaccine

14. **Which of the following is true for varicella vaccine?**
    A. Tuberculin skin testing (TST) should never be done on the same day that varicella vaccine is given
    B. Vaccinees pose a threat of shingles to other people in the same household
    C. It contains virus clearly different from the herpes simplex virus
    D. It should be avoided for 3 months after pregnancy

15. **Varicella vaccine**
    A. Is absolutely contraindicated for those living in close association with pregnant or symptomatic HIV+ people
    B. Should be used within 1 hour of re-constitution
    C. Is indicated in a non-immune person for up to 2 weeks after exposure to someone with varicella
    D. Seldom gives more than 50% protection

16. **Bacille Calmette-Guerin (BCG) vaccine is**
    A. Live attenuated *M. bovis*
    B. Live attenuated *M. tuberculosis*
    C. An extract from inactivated mycobacteria
    D. A conjugated polysaccharide derived from mycobacteria

17. **BCG vaccination and TB**
    A. Is more effective in adults than in children
    B. Is especially protective against pulmonary TB
    C. Appears to protect infants against miliary TB
    D. Is of no special benefit at any age

18. Which of the following is true for BCG vaccine?

A. It can be given simultaneously with most other vaccines
B. A booster dose is usual if the traveller is going to a really high-risk area
C. It is administered subcutaneously
D. The risk of TB for a traveller visiting >3 months becomes greater than the risk to the local residents

19. The most common adverse reaction to a BCG vaccination is

A. Painful local adenitis
B. Transient widespread pruritus
C. Local erythema and induration
D. Exacerbation of any underlying TB

20. Which of the following groups benefit most from BCG vaccination?

A. Immuno-compromised persons
B. HIV+ people
C. Asplenics
D. Those with a negative Mantoux test going as aid workers to Africa

21. BCG vaccine should be offered to otherwise suitable travellers going to

A. High-risk occupations overseas for >1 month
B. Areas for <1 month where multidrug-resistant TB (MDRTB) occurs
C. To Mantoux negative people going to developing countries for any period >1 month
D. Infants going from a low- to a high-risk country

22. A strongly positive Mantoux reaction in the potential traveller

A. Indicates active TB
B. Should be followed by active investigation for TB
C. Indicates previous exposure to leishmaniasis in a traveller who was born in an endemic area
D. Separates those who need BCG from those who do not

23. Purified protein derivative (PPD) 'conversion' is defined as

A. Absence of any skin reaction after re-testing at 6 months
B. Reduction in skin reaction to <5 mm over a 6-month period
C. A skin reaction >10 mm in someone who was previously a non-reactor or who showed a reaction <5 mm
D. A skin reactivity that goes from <5 mm to >5 mm induration in a 2-year period

24. Where there is a Mantoux 'conversion' (PPD conversion) in the returned traveller one should

A. Adopt a wait and see policy
B. Put the person in isolation until MDRTB is ruled out
C. Treat immediately with isoniazid (INH)
D. Start immediate triple therapy for 6–9 months

25. When doing a PPD test (Mantoux test) and giving a BCG

A. Avoid BCG if there has been a PPD test within the previous 4 weeks
B. PPD testing is contraindicated if the person has had a previous BCG
C. The interferon Y test should be used to help interpret doubtful PPD tests
D. Prior BCG vaccination should not influence interpretation of the PPD test

26. Cholera vaccine is

A. Best given by the parenteral route
B. Very effective by the oral route
C. Mandatory for entry to a small number of countries
D. Frequently associated with unpleasant side effects

27. The efficacy of oral cholera vaccine (OCV) is diminished if the subject

A. Takes an antacid medicine within 4 hours
B. Takes acetyl salicylic acid within 12 hours
C. Is on warfarin
D. Is taking chloroquin and/or proguanil

28. The efficacy of any OCV is diminished

A. If taken within 3 weeks of having had diarrhoea
B. In those of group O blood type
C. If given while the subject is on an oral antibiotic
D. If given at the same time as oral typhoid vaccine

29. Dukoral™ (killed cholera vaccine, KCV)

A. Gives excellent protection against classical 01 *V. cholera*
B. Is ineffective against *el Tor cholera*
C. Is very effective against *V. cholera 0139*
D. Offers little or no protection against enterotoxigenic *E. coli* (ETEC)

30. Diphtheria vaccine for adults and adolescents

A. Is known to interact unfavourably with parenteral typhoid Vi vaccine
B. Is more likely to give rise to systemic reactions in males than females
C. Must be given twice, 4 weeks apart, if there has been no primary course in the past
D. Needs to be given every 10 years if the subject travels to a high-risk area

31. The expected incidence of local reactions following a first tetanus 'booster' injection is up to

A. 10%
B. 25%
C. 35%
D. 40%

32. Tetanus or diphtheria immunization in travellers

A. Is not necessary in those over 75 years of age
B. Is contraindicated in the presence of an acute infection
C. Is dangerous to give to someone who has a proved hypersensitivity to penicillin in the past
D. May be dangerous when given to someone on immunosuppressive drugs

33. Which of the following is true for tetanus vaccination?

A. No more than five antitetanus shots should be given in a lifetime
B. Protective herd immunity by immunization determines the risk of tetanus outbreaks in any population
C. Any reaction to a first tetanus vaccination constitutes a contraindication to completion of the course
D. Severe reactions to tetanus vaccine usually indicate a high pre-existing antitoxin level

34. When giving measles vaccine for travel to developing countries

A. One dose should be given to travellers born since 1980
B. Two doses, 1 month apart, should be given to those born before 1970
C. Only give the vaccination to non-immunized persons who will be working in crowded places overseas
D. Assure your patient that measles vaccine is one of the safest vaccines on the market

35. The unpleasant taste of oral poliomyelitis vaccine (OPV, Sabin)

A. Is due to magnesium chloride
B. Is due to sodium chloride
C. Is due to thiomersal
D. Is due to polysorbate stabilizer

36. OPV contains

A. Thiomersal
B. Recombinant polio proteins
C. Live attenuated type 1, 2, and 3 polio virus
D. Killed whole-cell polio virus (all three types)

37. Which of the following fears is justified in relation to polio vaccine?

A. Inactivated parenteral polio vaccine (IPV) sometimes contains small amounts of simian virus-40 (SV40)
B. SV40-contaminated vaccine has been used in Western countries
C. SV40 is carcinogenic in humans
D. OPV may induce sterility in susceptible females

38. Vaccine-associated paralytic poliomyelitis (VAPP)

A. Has a characteristic symmetrical distribution
B. Is more likely to occur in children than in adults
C. Is estimated at about 0.5 to 3.5 in a million doses using OPV
D. Is estimated at about 1 in 20 million after IPV

39. Which of the following is true of VAPP?

A. VAPP occurs mostly after a first dose of OPV
B. VAPP is more likely to occur if the first dose was IPV
C. VAPP is more likely to occur if given on the same day as yellow fever vaccine
D. VAPP is more likely to occur if multiple parenteral injections have been given at the same time

40. Regarding OPV versus IPV

A. Both can cause VAPP
B. Immuno-compromised travellers should receive OPV rather than IPV
C. Both OPV and IPV need boosting every 10 years
D. Both result in polio-infected urine and/or faeces for 6 weeks

41. Which of the following is true of IPV?

A. IPV is more antigenic than OPV
B. IPV can be given to travelling infants within a few days of birth
C. IPV has an indefinite shelf-life if kept at 2–8°C
D. IPV is given in an adult dose to children >6 years old, even when combined with tetanus and diphtheria vaccine

42. Vero cell vaccines

A. Are free from added chemicals
B. Contain DNA-free particles of virus
C. Are developed in cells descended from the renal epithelium of monkeys
D. Match the pH and ionic composition of human extracellular fluid

43. Vero cell-derived Japanese encephalitis vaccine (Ixiaro®)

A. Is far more effective than mouse-brain-derived vaccine
B. Is suitable for people over 10 years of age
C. Contains aluminium hydroxide as an adjuvant
D. Is safe to give to a nursing mother

44. Which of the following is true of Ixiaro®?

A. Ixiaro® contains inactivated Japanese encephalitis virus strains SA 14-14-2
B. Ixiaro® confers protection for up to 5 years
C. Ixiaro® should be given in a course completed at least 48 hours before travel to an endemic area
D. Ixiaro® is normally given in three doses on days 0, 7, and 28

45. Which of the following is true for Ixiaro®?

A. A booster should be given every 5 years to maintain protection

B. It has a sub-optimal response if given subcutaneously

C. Adverse reactions occur in <1% of recipients

D. It is interchangeable with other Japanese encephalitis virus vaccines

46. Who should get Japanese encephalitis vaccine?

A. All travellers staying in endemic areas for >1 month

B. All elderly travellers to endemic areas

C. Child travellers to Mongolia

D. Visitors to urban areas in a Japanese encephalitis virus region

47. Rabies vaccine (human diploid cell vaccine, HDCV)

A. Is a cell-cultured live attenuated vaccine

B. Is a cell-cultured vaccine containing inactivated virus

C. Is a preparation of viral proteins derived from cell culture

D. Is a polysaccharide vaccine derived from culture on human diploid cells

48. Which of the following is true of HDCV rabies vaccine?

A. HDCV rabies vaccine may be given intravenously in acute situations

B. HDCV rabies vaccine should be injected into and around the bite area

C. The unopened freeze-dried vaccine deteriorates rapidly if kept at 16°C (approximately room temperature) for >2 hours

D. The dosage is the same for adults and children over 1 year old

49. Problems with the HDCV rabies vaccine include

A. Adverse reactions to albumin

B. Reduced response with concurrent use of mefloquine (lariam)

C. Ulceration of skin if given intradermally

D. Interaction with live vaccines

50. A traveller received two doses of purified vero cell-derived rabies vaccine (PVRV) in Germany 6 months ago. He is going next week to a high-risk area for rabies. You normally use HDCV. Should you

A. Restart the rabies schedule all over again, e.g. 0, 7, and 28 days

B. Give one dose of HDCV immediately and assume good cover

C. Order PVRV and give one dose before departure

D. Assume there is already sufficient cover from Germany

51. Which of the following is true for intradermal (ID) HDCV rabies versus IM routes?

A. ID gives lower antibody titres using the same time schedule (days 0, 7, and 28) as IM-administered vaccine

B. An ID schedule is less effective in the long term than an IM one

C. ID vaccine is less effective in post-exposure prophylaxis (PoEP) than IM vaccine

D. Five injections of ID vaccine are required (days 0, 3, 7, 14, and 28) compared to two IM injections (days 0 and 3) in post-exposure cases where the traveller has had full pre-exposure prophylaxis (PreEP) by either by the ID or the IM route

52. Rabies immune globulin (RIG)

A. Is always prepared from a human source

B. Should be given within 1 week of the bite

C. Should be given as early as possible in and around the wound

D. Should be given intravenously where it is certain the bite is from a rabid animal

53. The risk of rabies in the traveller is

A. Mainly from monkeys in Nepal

B. Greater in children than in adults

C. More likely from bats than from dogs in Thailand

D. Minimal from a quiet placid animal

54. Which of the following is true for rabies?

A. It is prevented by PreEP at days 0, 7, 21, or 28 when using a WHO-approved vaccine

B. It has a far higher overall death rate in adults than in children

C. Even 0.1 ml of WHO-approved vaccine ID confers immunity for a year

D. Deaths have been recorded after transplantation of organs from a rabies-infected donor

55. Routine non-conjugate pneumococcal vaccine for those who are 18 to 64 years old contains

A. Recombinant DNA

B. Inactivated whole cells

C. A mixture of purified capsular polysaccharides

D. Live attenuated organisms

56. Which of the following is true for pneumococcal vaccine (23-valent non-conjugated)?

A. One dose confers immunity for 10 years

B. It is used for those aged from 6 months upwards

C. It is recommended for transplant recipients

D. Cross-protection is provided against other capsulated organisms

57. **Pneumococcal vaccine (23-valent, non-conjugated) is recommended for all travellers**

    A. To reduce the chances of pneumonia
    B. Over 65 years of age
    C. To the 'meningitis belt' of Africa
    D. To the Hajj pilgrimage

58. **Influenza vaccine**

    A. Contains inactivated viruses of type A, B, and C influenza
    B. Contains inactivated type A virus only
    C. Is one of the few vaccines that can be stored at 0°C
    D. Contains traces of egg protein

59. **Influenza vaccine is a good option for travellers**

    A. Who are going from Cape Town to New York or London for the month of September
    B. Who are going from New York or London to Cape Town at Christmas time
    C. Who are breast feeding and going to the tropics for >2 months
    D. Aged >65 despite a *proved* history of allergy to mercury

60. **Influenza vaccine**

    A. Is slightly better than amantidine in preventing influenza
    B. Is more effective in older (>55 years) than in younger people
    C. Gives more local reactions if combined with an adjuvant
    D. Is contraindicated in children on long-term aspirin therapy

61. **Tick-borne encephalitis**

    A. Occurs in all continents
    B. Is hosted by wild and domestic animals as well as by humans
    C. Responds well to doxycycline in the early stages of the disease
    D. Is caused by a species of borrelia similar to that found in Lyme disease

62. **TBE vaccine, TicoVac (previously FSME-IMMUN)**

    A. Is an inactivated whole-cell virus vaccine
    B. Is a suspension of TBE virus subunits
    C. Is a live attenuated virus vaccine
    D. Is grown on human diploid cells

63. **Capsular polysaccharide vaccine against serogroups A, C, W-135, and Y (ACWY Vax, GlaxoSmithKline)**

    A. Should be given to all travellers going to sub-Saharan Africa for >1 month
    B. Should be given to all travellers going to Amazonia for >1 month
    C. Is particularly important in the dry season in Somalia
    D. Is approved for infants 6–12 months old

64. Conjugate quadrivalent meningitis vaccine

A. Affords limited protection against some other serotypes of N. meningitidis
B. Must be boosted every 2 years to ensure seroprotection
C. Is recommended for those going to Burkina Faso
D. Is now cheaper than the polysaccharide vaccine

65. The overall risk of an non-immunized traveller spending 6 months in a poor tropical country getting hepatitis A is

A. Greater than the chance of contracting influenza A or B
B. Greater than the chance of acquiring legionella
C. Greater than the chance of contracting malaria in West Africa
D. Greater than the chance of getting an animal bite with rabies risk

66. The hepatitis A vaccine most often used

A. Is a live attenuated suspension of hepatitis A virus (HAV)
B. Is a recombinant DNA vaccine
C. Is an inactivated vaccine prepared from HAV
D. Is considered absolutely safe in pregnancy

67. Neither Havrix™ (Glaxo Smith Kline) nor Avaxim™ (Sanofi Pasteur) should be given to people with known allergy to

A. Aluminium
B. Egg protein
C. Penicillin
D. Meningitis vaccine

68. One expects protective levels of anti-HAV antibodies in >80% of those who get one dose of Avaxim, Havrix, or VAQTA

A. After 2 weeks
B. After 4 weeks
C. After 12 weeks
D. After 18 weeks

69. Hepatitis B vaccine gives a less than expected response in

A. Those with bleeding disorders
B. Smokers
C. Non-athletes
D. Patients where there is simultaneous administration of HBV Ig

70. Which of the following are other risk factors for a sub-optimal response to hepatitis B vaccination?

A. Concurrent yellow fever vaccination
B. Subject taking mefloquine
C. Obesity
D. Known allergy to albumin

71. Hepatitis B vaccine should be *avoided* in

A. The immuno-compromised

B. Children under 1 year of age

C. The elderly (>70 years)

D. Lactation and/or pregnancy

72. Hepatitis B vaccine has been linked to

A. Chronic fatigue syndrome (CFS)

B. Multiple sclerosis (MS)

C. Parkinson's disease

D. Sudden infant death syndrome (SIDS)

73. Hepatitis B vaccine

A. Offers some protection against hepatitis E

B. Contains surface and core antigens of hepatitis B virus (HBV)

C. Should be given routinely to anyone diagnosed with hepatitis C

D. Is given in adult dosage to those over 6 years of age

74. Seroprotection after vaccination against hepatitis B means that there is more than a designated value of

A. Antibody to HBc antigen in the subject's blood

B. Antibody to HBs antigen in the subject's blood

C. Antibody to HBe antigen in the subject's blood

D. All three antibodies in the subject's blood

75. After an accelerated schedule (0, 7, and 21 days) of hepatitis B vaccine

A. Approximately 1% of *healthy individuals* fail to achieve an adequate antibody response

B. Seroprotection is never achieved

C. Seroprotection occurs in < 60% of recipients after 1 year

D. Seroprotection occurs in > 90% of recipients after 1 year

76. Which of the following is true for heptitis B vaccination?

A. It requires at least one booster after the primary course to ensure long-term (>40 years) immunity in immunocompetent people

B. The non-responder rate to conventional hepatitis B vaccines is greater in children than in adults

C. It is unlikely to reduce the incidence of hepatocellular carcinoma

D. It confers immunocompetence against hepatitis B if anti-HBsAG >5 IU/ml

77. Combined hepatitis A and B vaccination

A. Gives somewhat less protection than administration of the two vaccines separately

B. Gives more severe local reactions than either hepatitis A or hepatitis B vaccine separately

C. Can be used as a long-life booster against hepatitis A instead of the monodose hepatitis A

D. Needs at least three injections to elicit maximum immunity

78. Hepatitis B immunoglobulin (500 IU for adults)

A. Is always used in conjunction with hepatitis A immunoglobulin

B. Is found in good amounts in pooled human immuoglobulin in developed countries

C. Is a useful pre-exposure injection in certain travellers

D. Is recommended for specific non-immune travellers to very high-risk areas

79. Which of the following is true when comparing single vaccines for hepatitis A (Avaxim™) and Havrix™?

A. There is a significant difference in immunogenicity

B. There is a considerable difference in price

C. More local reactions occur after Avaxim™

D. Havrix™ elicits a more rapid and higher response than Avaxim™

80. Which of the following is true when comparing combined vaccines for hepatitis A and typhoid, and the monovalent vaccines?

A. There is better immunogenicity with single vaccines

B. The hepatitis A component of the combined vaccine interferes with the immunogenicity of the typhoid component

C. More local reactions occur after the combined vaccine

D. There is equal tolerability between the combined and single vaccines

81. Parenteral typhoid vaccine (Vi)

A. Is a live attenuated vaccine

B. Protects against S. typhi and S. paratyphi

C. Retains efficacy if exposed to temperatures >30°C for 24 hours

D. Is suitable for children over 6 months of age

82. Which of the following are contraindications to giving parenteral typhoid vaccine?

A. Tetracyclines

B. Mefloquine

C. Acute febrile illness

D. Intradermal rabies in the same arm

83. One can expect injectable Vi vaccine to have maximum protective efficacy against S. typhi after

A. 3 months

B. 6 months

C. 3 years

D. 6 years

84. Oral typhoid vaccine

A. Is a suspension of purified Vi antigen
B. Is a suspension of whole-cell inactivated S. *typhi*
C. Is a suspension of whole-cell inactivated S. typhi and selected strains of S. paratyphi
D. Is a suspension of live attenuated mutant S. *typhi*

85. Which of the following is true for oral typhoid vaccine (US schedule, four capsules on alternate days)?

A. Protection starts about 1 week after the final dose
B. Protection is about 50% 10 years after the course
C. It can be used in children >3 years of age
D. More secure absorption occurs if the capsule is broken open and the contents taken with a hot drink

86. When using oral typhoid capsules one should

A. Increase the dose for immunocompromised persons
B. Advise the subject not to eat for 2 hours afterwards
C. Repeat the whole series if the subject misses one dose
D. Take special care with subjects' stools in case S. *typhi* infects other members of the household

87. Modern human immunoglobulin (HIG) preparations

A. Give less protection against HAV at 2 weeks than active immunization
B. May transmit hepatitis C
C. May transmit HIV
D. Are certain to prevent fulminant hepatitis A if given in adequate dose before travelling

88. Which of these vaccines is a live attenuated preparation?

A. Anthrax vaccine
B. Plague vaccine
C. Lyme
D. Varicella vaccine

89. Which of the following vaccines need a booster dose some years after the primary schedule is completed?

A. Typhim Vi
B. Quadrivalent meningitis vaccine (non-conjugated)
C. Rabies HDCV vaccine
D. Pneumococcal polysaccharide vaccine

90. Plague vaccine

    A. Is a live attenuated vaccine

    B. Is effective after one dose

    C. Gives adequate protection for 2 years

    D. Has had little controlled study

91. A man of 65 is planning to work in Angola as an agricultural advisor for a year. In addition to the regular travel vaccines which of the following would you advise him to receive?

    A. Pertussis vaccine

    B. Pertussis and zoster vaccines

    C. Varicella vaccine

    D. Anthrax vaccine

General vaccinology

1. D. Skeletal muscle is more vascular than subcutaneous fat, thus antigen is absorbed, mobilized, and processed more quickly after an IM injection than after an SC injection. The SC route has been associated with response failure to hepatitis B, rabies, and influenza vaccine. Subcutaneous fat is richly innervated and so SC injections are more painful than IM ones. Local reactions are more common after SC injections because subcutaneous tissue has a richer lymphatic supply than muscle. Note that a 26-gauge needle is too small for IM injections in an adult.

2. C. The IM route is used to avoid delayed local reactions after potentially irritating adjuvant-containing and large volume vaccines. The SC route is preferred for most live vaccines which will be more slowly absorbed from this site. Use the SC route if there is a bleeding tendency, e.g. if the patient is on warfarin. If the IM route must be used in these patients, e.g. with hepatitis B vaccine, then use a small bore needle and apply pad pressure for some minutes afterwards.

3. C. Active immunization implies administration of live (attenuated) or killed (inactivated) whole organisms or modified parts of such organisms, e.g. tetanus toxoid. Active immunization evokes a B-cell or B-cell and T-cell response in the subject. Active immunization can be enteral or parenteral.

4. D. The rare tragedy of a recipient acquiring the disease from a live vaccine, whether due to back mutation or a wrong dose or impaired resistance or a combination of all three, is a nightmare scenario. The classic example is vaccine-associated paralytic poliomyelitis due to live oral polio vaccine (Sabin vaccine). Immunogenicity after live vaccines involves both humoral cell (B-cell) and long-term memory cell (T-cell) responses. Thus even one fully immunogenic dose can confer immunity for many years, perhaps life. Oral administration makes many live vaccines very attractive but also poses the problem of releasing live organisms into the sewage system and creates the possibility of direct cross-transmission. Although specific levels of antibody in the serum are assumed to indicate immuno-protection, that is, someone with these levels is protected from the disease, this concept is open to debate. For example, it appears that there is no specific protective level of anti-pertussis antibodies. Idiosyncratic individual response may play an important role in determining resistance to antigen assault.

5. B. Killed vaccines need adjuvants such as aluminium or biodegradable biospheres to improve their antigenicity. Although they usually stimulate both humoral and cellular immune systems, they need repeated administration. In general, during the primary schedule, it is acceptable to give the next dose up to 4 days before the minimum recommended date. Rabies vaccine is an exception to this rule.

The great advantage of inactivated vaccines is their high safety profile and their inability to multiply or revert to pathogenicity in the recipient.

6. A. Conjugate vaccines involve the conjugation of a weak bacterial polysaccharide antigen with a protein, thus enhancing immunogenicity. This conjugation converts T-cell independent carbohydrate antigen into a T-cell dependent antigen, with all the associated benefits in terms of immunological response. Conjugate vaccines are of great advantage in the young (<2 years old), where there is little immune response to carbohydrate antigens.

Recall that meningococci, pneumococci and haemophilus influenza type B (Hib) are all coated by a polysaccharide capsule. Success in conjugate vaccines started with Hib—the most common cause of bacterial meningitis—and has been followed by meningococcus serotype C, pneumococcus, and quadrivalent meningococcus.

7. A. There appears to be no risk of either increased adverse reactions or immunogenic interference with concomitant administration.

One should not withold giving a conjugate and non-conjugate vaccine at the same time in special circumstances, e.g. the last-minute traveller.

8. C. Protein carriers render the vaccination far more immunogenic and even induce immunity in children under 2 years. Unconjugated polysaccharide vaccines are not boosted by subsequent doses; one starts from scratch each time. To boost a vaccine means repeating the vaccine so that it stimulates T-cells that have a memory of the initial dose. There is no long-term or initial memory when giving an unconjugated polysaccharide vaccine.

9. A. Restarting the series after missing a dose is a major disadvantage of giving live oral typhoid vaccine (Ty21a).

10. D. The subject may well be misinformed and the alleged allergic reaction in the past may have been due to some other antibiotic. Traces of neomycin and other antibiotics may be found in many vaccines, e.g. IPV and rabies vaccine, and so one should take extra care when giving them in this case. Nonetheless the amounts are so small that hypersensitivity reactions are unlikely to occur or are confined locally. No currently recommended vaccine contains penicillin. Preservatives, including thimerosal (mercury), are being eliminated from all vaccines, including meningococcal polysaccharide vaccine.

11. A. Traces of egg protein are found in the following vaccines: measles, mumps, rabies,TBE, influenza, and yellow fever. When giving these vaccines a test dose of 0.1 ml should be given intradermally if the patient says he or she has an allergy to eggs.

12. A. An urticarial pruritic rash is most likely to be a simple allergic response to an unknown allergen. If this is the first time the person has been exposed to this allergen then the response is, strictly speaking, an anaphylactoid reaction. A severe allergic reaction encompasses pruritic rash, angioedema (often of lips, eyes, and tongue), dyspnoea, tachycardia, and cough.

True anaphylactic shock is a worsening of the above with laryngeal oedema, inspiratory stridor, wheeze, substernal pain, hypotension, and collapse. Such problems generally occur very quickly after exposure to the allergen, usually within 10 minutes.

A vasovagal attack (simple faint) may occur if the patient is injected while in the erect position (very rarely if sitting). It is unlikely that any experienced medic will mistake this for a more sinister reaction.

13. A. Adrenaline should always be on hand and given as a priority. The adult dose is 0.5 ml (500 µg) IM of a 1:1000 solution. Repeat once after about 5 minutes in the absence of clinical improvement or if consciousness remains impaired as a result of hypotension. Chlorpheniramine

10 mg can be given slowly IV as can hydrocortisone 100–200 mg IV. Life-threatening anaphylaxis is rare (frequency varies from 1/45,000 to 1/100,000). It is important to place the patient in the shock position, administer oxygen, and find IV access as soon as possible.

Specific vaccines

1. A. Tetanus vaccine should always be considered in a routine pre-travel consultation but only given when indicated. Consensus, especially in the UK, suggests that, while five tetanus injections is normally sufficient for a lifetime, extra ones may be given if there is a high level of risk. Reactions are more likely the more often the vaccine is given. About one quarter of all travellers are not completely immunized against tetanus.

Tetanus quick sticks (TQS) or tetanus dipsticks take 10 minutes to read and are 100% specific for tetanus antibodies. If the test is positive, one can assume protection against tetanus for at least 5 years. Sensitivity is about 55% for titres of 0.01 IU/ml but can be taken as 100% at levels of >0.5 IU/ml, which is five times greater than the accepted protective limit of 0.1 IU/ml. Automated tetanus antibody immunity testing (Avecon Diagnostics) is able to process 800 tests per hour and has a sensitivity limit of 0.01 IU/ml.

2. A. Hajj and Umrah pilgrims are required to have a certificate of vaccination against serotypes ACYW135 at least 10 days and not more than 3 years prior to arrival in Saudia. This is because of outbreaks of W135 during recent pilgrimages. Ideally one should use the conjugate quadrivalent vaccine for visits to any high-risk country.

3. D. Yellow fever vaccine is a live vaccine and is contraindicated in children <9 months for fear of YFVA-ND (see below). It is also contraindicated in pregnancy (unless there is an overriding risk of yellow fever), in the immunocompromised, in those with thymus disorders, and in those with severe egg allergy.

Protection is probably life-long although International Certification is required every 10 years.

Different live vaccines should be given on the same day or otherwise separated by 3–4 weeks because of the risk of a reduced response.

4. D. Angola is a yellow fever endemic country. Proof of vaccination is required in all those who enter who are over 1 year of age.

5. C. Paraguay, where it abuts Argentina, has recently experienced yellow fever and vaccination is recommended (WHO, 2011). The WHO and CDC maps of yellow fever-affected countries are now identical. Many countries in Africa and in South and Central America are affected, although often outbreaks are erratic and unpredictable. Although Zambia and South Africa are both officially declared yellow fever free (WHO) they can demand proof of yellow fever vaccination even if the arriving passenger has ony transited in the airport of a yellow fever endemic country. There is no convincing explanation for the absence of clinical yellow fever in Asia. Most major cities in the American tropics and much of tropical Asia now harbour *Aedes aegypti*. Note that India considers Zambia to be an area of risk of yellow fever transmission (Travax, 2012).

6. D. The 10-day requirement only applies to the first dose of vaccine. Live vaccines should be given at the same session or separated by 4 weeks. Most yellow fever vaccine-related deaths occur in the elderly (>65 years). If there is no skin reaction to a test dose then you can give the remainder 10–15 minutes later.

7. B. YFV-ND occurs mainly in those aged <9 months.Thus it is most common after a first immunization. Neurotropic disease has a mortality of 6%, not as high as with the viscerotropic variety. Both have an incubation period of 4–23 days. CNS signs, fever, headache, and CSF pleocytosis occur. Some cases have now been reported in adults. One estimation puts the risk at <1 per 8 million recipients. There have been <35 cases documented since 1945. The live attenuated 17D strain developed in the 1930s is still the only vaccine used. Infants 6–9 months old may be only vaccinated in special circumstances, e.g. during major outbreaks.

8. A. YFVA-VD is well authenticated. It has been recognized since 2001 when the first 7 cases were reported. Multiple organ failure occurs within 4–23 days after vaccination and yellow fever virus abounds in the blood. It reaches figures of 20 per million doses in those over 60 years. Unfortunately yellow fever virus has a fatality rate of over 60% in that age group in whom it can occur in 1/50,000 of first-time vaccinees. Problems with the thymus but not with the thyroid appear to increase the risk of multiorgan failure following vaccination. It is proposed that YFVA-DA is more common in the elderly because there is a longer post-vaccination viraemia due to a reduced immune response in older people. YFVA-ND and YFVA-VD (viscerotropic disease) were first reported in the *Lancet* in 2001.

9. B. Do not give vaccines to a febrile patient. Yellow fever vaccine is not contraindicated in the other options provided care is taken. Many give yellow fever vaccine to HIV+ asymptomatic patients provided the CD4 count is over 200 cells/ml. Remember the CD4 count may be down for some other immunological reason. A report from Buenos Aires showed that a value over 300 (range 306–1300) was without incident in a series of HIV+ patients. However, it is recommended that yellow fever vaccine be withheld from symptomatic HIV+ patients, especially if febrile. Most alleged egg allergies are not true allergies at all. If such a patient has been vaccinated against yellow fever within 20 years, re-vaccination should be omitted as one can be confident that immunity still persists. Where there is genuine fear of egg allergy one should give 0.1 ml of the vaccine ID and if there is no reaction after 30 minutes it is safe to give the remaining 0.4 ml SC. There is evidence that even 0.1 ml ID provides seroprotection.

10. D. Concurrent administration of BCG and yellow fever vaccine may cause difficulty in interpreting a later PPD skin test because of the possibility of live virus interaction. Usual doses of chloroquin or mefloquine do not interfere with yellow fever vaccine response.

It was thought desirable to separate oral typhoid and yellow fever vaccination by 3 weeks because some studies showed an impaired response to both with concurrent administration. However, it is now held that Ty21a can be administered simultaneously with or at any interval before or after any other injectable live vaccine (WHO, 2011).

11. D. MPSV4 is a freeze-dried non-conjugated polysaccharide vaccine containing 50 μg of polysaccharide from each of the four strains. One 0.5 ml dose protects for 3–5 years. Store the prefilled syringe in a fridge (2–8°C), where it will remain stable for 3 years. Use within 2 hours of reconstitution. Quadrivalent vaccines have now replaced the bivalent (A and C) preparation. The multivalent polysaccharide vaccines available are Menomune (Sanofi), Mencevac (Glaxo Smith Kline), and ACWYvax (Glaxo Smith Kline). MPSV4 is used in the preferred choice of vaccine for those over 55 years (CDC). It can be given to children as young as 9 months but does not stimulate T-cell immunity, gives no mucosal immunity, and is less and less effective with repeated doses.

12. C. Meningococcal conjugate vaccine (MCV4) is approved for use in those aged 2–55 years of age. In one study, in children under 4 years of age, efficacy fell from 90% to less than 10% at 3 years. The vaccine is not recommended for those <2 years because of poor immunogenicity, although infants older than 6 months may show a satisfactory response to the serogroup A component. It is as immunogenic as non-conjugate vaccines and has the great advantage of reducing nasopharyngeal carriage of *Neisseria meningitidis* (mucosal immunity). Newer conjugate vaccines are being developed which have the potential of protecting infants <2 years but are not in general use yet. This is important because infants experience the highest rate of invasive meningococcal disease and also have the highest mortality rate. Examples of MCV4 include Menveo® (Novartis) and Menactra® (Sanofi).

13. A. Varicella vaccine is a live attenuated viral vaccine. It is recommended for those travellers over 13 years of age who are likely to have close contact with local populations. It is given in two doses, 4–8 weeks apart. Like all live vaccines it is contraindicated in pregnancy and in immunocompromised people. Adsorbed anthrax vaccine is given in six doses: 0, 2, and 4 weeks followed by 6, 12, and 18 months. It was given widely to US soldiers in the first Gulf War. It is a restricted vaccine and its efficacy is not certain. Pneumococcal vaccine contains polysaccharides from 23 pneumococcal serotypes and is widely used in elderly, asplenic, and immunocompromised travellers.

14. D. Varicella vaccine should not be given during pregnancy, during lactation, and until 3 months after pregnancy ends. Women should also avoid pregnancy during the course (Travax, 2012). Up to 90% of adult travellers are already protected by a primary attack but in the remaining 10% the vaccine is recommended, especially for children and for all making extended visits overseas. Varicella can be a serious illness in adults and even in chidren.

Zoster (shingles) is a reactivation of dormant virus in the dorsal root ganglia, usually in the elderly and, more often nowadays, in immunocompromised or stressed people of all ages.

Simultaneous tuberculin skin testing poses no threat nor is the live virus excreted in the faeces, in contrast to OPV.

Varicella-zoster virus is morphologically identical to herpes simplex virus.

15. B. For optimal efficacy varicella vaccine should be used immediately or at least 1 hour after reconstitution. Many hold that vaccinees pose no threat even living in close contact with pregnant or immunocompromised individuals. Nonetheless, it is prudent that vaccine recipients should avoid close contact with these high-risk groups for 6 weeks following vaccination. This is especially so if the recipients develop a rash, which may be infective, after vaccination.

Varicella vaccine is effective in preventing or in modifying disease severity when given up to 5 days after exposure to varicella. Protective efficacy is in the region of 97–99% after a second dose. Varicella zoster immune globulin (VGIG) may be used for up to 5 days after exposure of non-immune subjects in a high-risk situation. Storage temperature depends on vaccine formulation and may differ in different regions, e.g. the USA, Canada, and Europe. Both Varivax (Sanofi) and Varilrix (Glaxo Smith Kline) should be stored at +2 to +8°C. The lysophilized vaccine should be stored in a deep freeze (−50°C to −15°C). All varicella vaccines should be used immediately after reconstitution. The quadrivalent Proquad vaccine developed by Merck has been discontinued.

16. A. BCG vaccine is live attenuated *M. bovis*. In many countries it is given shortly after birth. It is not given as a routine childhood vaccination in the USA.

Apart from TB, BCG has been used, with conflicting claims, to protect against or ameliorate such diverse conditions as leprosy, Buruli ulcer, multiple sclerosis and Parkinson's disease.

17. C. BCG appears to be most useful in protecting infants under 1 year old against extrapulmonary and miliary TB. In the UK it is reckoned to be 80% effective in protecting against TB in children at high risk. It gives no useful protection against pulmonary TB. BCG vaccination is only offered to infants in the UK in communities with an average incidence of TB of at least 40 per 100,000 and to unvaccinated individuals who come from, or whose parents or grandparents come from, countries where the incidence exceeds 40 per 100,000.

BCG is sometimes given to travellers deemed at high risk from TB when the PPD test is negative.

Unfortunately guidelines on the use of BCG in travel medicine are not uniform.

18. A. BCG can be given simultaneously with most other vaccines, including all the usual childhood ones. The WHO does not recommend a 'booster'. The vaccine is given intradermally. It is likely that after 3 months the traveller runs the same risk of acquiring TB as the local population.

19. C. Local erythema and induration is not considered a serious adverse reaction. Unfortunately the site may break down and any ensuing ulceration is slow to heal. Very occasionally this is severe enough to warrant skin grafting. Although severe disease is unusual, it is a possible complication of BCG vaccination. Care must be taken to use vaccine that is at the right dilution and in date, and to give it correctly.

20. D. Those with a negative Mantoux test who will be working closely with people who have open TB should be considered for BCG vaccination. However, this only applies to a minority of travellers. Those with conditions such as HIV, on immunosuppressant drugs, with lymphoma, leukaemia, Hodgkin's disease, or currently on systemic steroids or other immunosuppressant drugs and those who are pregnant should not receive any live vaccine. A negative Mantoux test must be taken in conjunction with the patient's history, including when, where, and how the test was given and who read it.

21. D. WHO guidelines suggest that BCG be offered to infants going from low-risk to high-risk regions. Clearly the individual practitioner must make this decision after informed discussion with the parent/guardian. Common practice involves skin testing before and after travel and then giving appropriate treatment if the test 'converts'. The practice of giving preventative treatment, e.g. INH, to anyone at high-risk, e.g. health workers, is hotly contested.

22. B. The Manotux test is considered positive if there is an induration >10 mm 72 hours after ID injection of 5 IU of PPD delivered in 0.1 ml. It is generally positive in active TB. It is sometimes weakly positive in leishmaniasis (cross-reaction). False positives and negatives are common, the latter especially in the immunocompromised. The need for anti-TB treatment is based on history, physical examination, and laboratory tests, e.g. acid fast bacilli in sputum, raised erythrocyte sedimentation rate (ESR), and suspicious chest X-ray (CXR).

Note that any of the options given may be true, with 22B being the best choice.

23. D. Conversion from no reactivity to reactivity, after immune challenge by PPD, is presumptive evidence of active TB unless proved otherwise. However, once conversion occurs some physicians would first do a CXR and if this is negative the person is put on INH 300 mg QID for 6–12 months along with vitamin B6 50 mg po QID. The patient is monitored for any sign of active TB, which, if found, is treated aggressively. If the CXR is positive or doubtful then full anti-TB treatment is started.

24. C. One adopts the same policies outlined in the last answer. Some authorities recommend a two-step Mantoux test for travellers who have spent >6 months in a high-risk area. In this method, if the first test is negative in 48–72 hours, the test is repeated in approximately 2 weeks.

Nowadays most will do the more expensive but more reliable quantaferon test (see next question).

25. C. This is probaby the best answer although option B is widely held, especially in the USA. Most agree that BCG should never be given to a person who has a strongly positive tuberculin skin test (Mantoux test). The current interferon test is more specific for TB antigen than the earlier interferon test. It is particularly helpful in identifying latent tuberculosis.

26. B. Oral cholera vaccine, e.g. Dukoral™ (formalin and heat-inactivated vibrio), is very effective and has almost no adverse side effects. Since 1992 cholera vaccination has no longer been officially required for entry to any country but it is still demanded in certain careers, e.g. some merchant seamen. Dukoral™ contains the recombinant B-subunit of the cholera toxin plus killed *V. cholerae* O1 (Inaba and Ogawa serotypes and El Tor and classical biotypes).

27. D. The efficacy of live OCVs is diminished if taken within a week of chloroquin, proguanil, or antibiotics. However, neither mefloquine nor antacids appear to interfere nor does yellow fever vaccination. Although it has been demonstrated in the past that live OCVs do not remain viable in the intestine long enough to be strongly antigenic, newer live OCVs, e.g. Orochol-E, have protective efficacy and a single dose is sometimes given to healthcare workers after an outbreak starts.

28. C. Most oral antibiotics kill the cholera vibrio and so reduce or abolish the immunogenicity of a live OCV. Group O individuals are more susceptible to acquiring cholera than others but respond as favourably to oral vaccine. Avoid food and drink 1 hour before and after taking any OCV. Efficacy is diminished by the acid secretions provoked so taking antacids may be advantageous. There is no strong evidence to show that the efficacy of the vaccine is diminished by oral typhoid vaccine, by simultaneous yellow fever immunization, or by recent diarrhoea. Normally adults take two doses separated by 1 week and children <6 years old take three doses with similar intervals.

29. A. A KCV, e.g. Dukoral™, is up to 90% effective against classical and El Tor cholera for the first 6 months. Immunity starts after 3 weeks. No vaccine protects against 0139 cholera, a type first described in India in 1992. Type 0139 is still responsible for severe outbreaks in India and Bangladesh. KCV may provide protection (50–60%) against ETEC as both share similar β-subgroups. One study on 11,000 >2-year-olds in Mozambique showed a dramatic fall in both cholera and ETEC when prophylactic Dukoral was given. A vaccine obtained by using antibodies in the colostrum of dairy cattle shows better promise in preventing ETEC.

Newer bivalent OCVs, e.g. Shanchol or mORCVAX, show great promise since they incorporate serotype 0139. They are now targated at high-risk children aged ≥1 year whereas Dukoral is only given to those ≥2 years. Significant protection from current cholera vaccines is 2 years (WHO).

30. D. Diphtheria outbreaks have been reported in the former USSR and more recently in the Balkans, where herd immunity has fallen dramatically. Each 0.5 ml dose contains 4 IU of purified diphtheria toxoid. There are no known interactions with other medicinal products but systemic reactions occasionally occur, especially in those who have received repeated doses. A primary schedule consists of three doses each separated by at least 4 weeks. In the USA the third dose is delayed for 6–12 months. Fifty per cent of UK adults over 30 years old are susceptible to diphtheria.

The combination vaccine (Td/IPV), containing reduced-dose diphtheria component, should be used in adults (over 10 years) for both primary courses and boosters (Travax, 2012). The high-dose diphtheria toxoid used in children is denoted by capital D.

31. A. The rate of local reactions (pain, swelling, redness) is about 1 in 10 rising to 50–80% with further doses of tetanus toxoid.

32. B. Acute infection is a contraindication to all immunizations. Sixty per cent of 70-year-olds have little or no immunity to tetanus/diphtheria. There is no penicillin in the vaccine. Immunosuppressed people give a suboptimal response and may need another dose. Travellers should be off immunosuppressant drugs for 3 months to regain full immunogenicity. In the UK tetanus toxoid for adults is only given as a component of combination vaccines, e.g. Revaxis (tetanus, diphtheria, polio).

33. D. Normally five tetanus shots in a lifetime are sufficient. However, an extra shot should be given if 10 years has elapsed since the last one and the traveller is going to a high-risk area/job. Unlike diphtheria, herd immunity does not apply to tetanus, where the object of the immunization is to provide individual protection.

The only absolute contraindication to completing a course of tetanus shots is confirmed anaphylaxis. Severe reactions are usually indicative of high antitoxin levels due to repeated immunization. The UK 2012 updates on tetanus shots refines the recommendations into 'sometimes advised', which is essentially to have a shot if a suspect injury occurs, and 'usually advised', if the traveller has not had a tetanus shot in the previous 10 years.

34. B. It is best to consult a standard table relating the year of birth to the requirement for none, one, or two (3 months apart) MMR shots. Since 1970 measles has been incorporated into the childhood vaccination schedule of most developed countries. Thus two doses of the vaccine are given to travellers born before 1970, although most will have already have acquired immunity. Only one dose is given to those born after 1970. The disease is easily caught, can be very serious, and is widespread in the developing world. The fall-off in vaccination in developed countries, and the re-introduction of the measles virus from overseas, has meant a serious recrudescence of measles in North America, Israel, Japan, and many European countries. MMR (measles/mumps/rubella) vaccine can be given at any age. Measles vaccine is a live vaccine and although it can have serious adverse effects, ranging from a mild rash to encephalitis, the dangers associated with the illness greatly outweigh those of vaccination. Measles is highly communicable and appears to have been transmitted recently from person-to-person on a flight from Frankfurt to Barcelona (both returning from developing countries).

35. A. MgCl$_2$ (>200 mg/ml) gives OPV a bitter metallic taste. Giving the vaccine on a sugar lump or with a syrup can mask this but OPV should not be given with general foodstuffs that contain preservatives.

36. C. OPV is a highly effective live attenuated vaccine containing types 1, 2, and 3 polio virus. It may contain minute traces of neomycin, streptomycin, and penicillin.

37. B. In the 1960s SV40 was found in IPV that had been prepared using kidney cells of rhesus monkeys. Up to 30 million Americans received SV40-contaminated IPV between 1955 and 1963. Athough there is nothing to suggest that SV40 is carcinogenic in humans, it may cause tumours in rodents and is found in diverse human cancers, including lymphomas. Reports that polio vaccine may transmit HIV/AIDS or be a cause of sterility have no factual basis. The dream that polio would be eliminated by 2000 has proved illusory. Huge immunization schemes with OPV are underway in India (2012).

38. C. VAPP occurs only after OPV with an estimated risk of 0.5–3.5 per million doses. It is more likely to occur in adults than in children. VAPP figures vary widely in the literature. Makers of OPV state 'the risk is rare, is mainly associated with type 3 component' and 'relates primarily to adults not previously immunised'. Since 1999 only IPV is used in the USA and many other countries have since followed suit. VAPP is identical to clinical polio caused by wild type polio virus. Both have an asymmetrical distribution of paralysis.

39. A. According to WHO the risk of VAPP is greater after the first than after subsequent doses. If it occurs after subsequent doses it is irrelevant if the first dose was IPV or OPV. Theoretically muscle damage, e.g. by multiple intramuscular injections, may predispose to VAPP, but this is not proved.

40. C. A booster dose every 10 years is recommended for both OPV and IPV. The rare risk of VAPP after OPV has caused IPV to be the vaccine of choice in developed countries, but OPV is far cheaper, can be given easily and quickly in an outbreak, and is very effective. OPV is a live vaccine and should not be given to pregnant or immunocompromised patients. Ideally all non-immunized members of a household should be vaccinated if OPV is given to one member because the live polio virus is present in the faeces for 6 weeks and cross-contamination can occur if hygiene standards are lax. There is also the danger of vaccine-derived polio virus entering sewage systems with unknown consequences as regards spread and mutation. This problem is not present with IPV.

41. D. The 'adult' dose of the triple vaccine is given >6 years of age. This contains low-dose diphtheria. Neither IPV nor OPV should be given <6–8 weeks of age. IPV has a shelf-life of 3 years even if kept in the refrigerator. OPV is more antigenic than IPV. OPV confers intestinal immunity, most probably for life. IPV is far more expensive than OPV. Revaxis (TdIPV) contains the low dose of diphtheria toxoid suitable for adults (small 'd'). Remember that primary combined vaccinations that protect against diphtheria, tetanus, pertussis, and poliomyelitis are available from infancy to childhood, e.g. Pediacel and Infanrix. Repavax is suitable for all ages from 3 years upwards.

42. C. Vero cells are cell lineages derived from renal epithelial cells of an African green monkey in Japan in 1962. Organisms such as the rabies virus or trypanosomes can be cultured in them. The vero cell lineage does not show senescence. The word 'vero' is an acronym of 'verdo reno' (green kidney).

43. C. Ixiaro contains aluminium hydroxide as an adjuvant. It gives seroprotection >95% at 6 months and >84% at 12 months. This is slightly better than that achieved by previous vaccines derived from living organisms, e.g. JE-VAC. Currently it is only recommended in those over 17 years of age. It has not been tested in pregnancy or in breast-feeding mothers.

44. A. Ixiaro® contains the strains mentioned. Aluminium hydroxide and protamine sulphate are also present, but there are no stabilizers, e.g. gelatine or lactalbumin. Protection lasts around 1 year. A course consists of two injections 28 days apart and should be completed at least 1 week before departure. This is because seroconversion has been observed to rise from 29.4% 10 days after the first vaccination to 97.3% 1 week after the second vaccination.

45. B. It should be given by the IM route for the best response. A booster dose is recommended every 2–3 years but should be given every year in those at special risk, e.g. laboratory workers. Adverse reactions occur in about 40% of recipients and are usually mild in nature (myalgia, headache). It is probably unwise to complete a course of Japanese encephalitis virus immunization with a vaccine derived by a different method.

46. A. Consider vaccination for repeated visits to or prolonged stays in endemic areas. Do not neglect infants and children who, like the elderly and the immunocompromised, are more likely to get serious disease. Even short stays in rural parts can pose a risk, particularly during epidemics. Such outbreaks often follow the start of the rainy season, when mosquito activity is maximal. Japanese encephalitis has not been reported from Mongolia. Apart from the military, few cases have been reported in travellers. Overall, the risk of acquiring Japanese encephalitis while travelling in Asia is extremely low. However, the risk for an individual traveller is highly variable and depends on factors such as the season, location and duration of travel, and the activities of the person. The charitable organization Programme for Appropriate Technology in Health (PATH) is currently involved in immunizing children in India.

47. B. HDCV is prepared as a freeze-dried powder derived from the Wistar rabies strain and is inactivated with β-propiolactone. After reconstitution with water the vaccine should be used as soon as possible. Neural derived vaccine, available in India, should not be used because of reported serious complications. Excellent vaccines containing inactivated virus grown on purified vero cells (PVRV), e.g. Verorab, and inactivated virus grown on purified chick embryo cells (PCEC) are also available in some countries. You MUST check with the manufacturers' recommendations when using a rabies vaccine

48. D. The vaccine appears to be safe even to an under 1-year-old. Never give rabies vaccine IV or into a wound. The IM route (deltoid in adult, anterolateral thigh in child) is recommended by the manufacturers. They do not recommend the ID route but 0.1 ml ID is accepted practice in many countries. The freeze-dried vaccine retains potency of >2.5 IU even if exposed to 37°C for a month.

49. A. Very rarely there may be a reaction to the albumin (50 mg/ml) in HDCV. The use of purified vero cell rabies vaccine (PVRV), purified duck embryo vaccine (PDEV) and purified chick embryo vaccine (PCEV) helps to obviate this. If chromatographically purified rabies vaccine (CPRV) becomes available the risk will be minimal.

Concurrent use of chloroquine may possibly interfere with the response to ID rabies vaccine. Ulceration of the skin will only occur if there is faulty technique or infection is introduced unwittingly.

There is no contraindication to concurrent administration of a live vaccine.

50. B. Lengthening the intervals between rabies shots is acceptable while shortening them is not. HDCV is interchangeable with PVRV.

51. A. There is a greater anitibody response to IM than to ID rabies vaccine but seroprotection is achieved by either. Either a two-dose schedule of ID vaccine (0.1 ml) or preferably a two-dose schedule of the IM vaccine (1.0 ml) is appropriate PoEP if the traveller has had a full PreEP. A better anamnestic response may be achieved by a four-site ID post-exposure at a one-off visit. A 5-day post-exposure course is required in the unprotected, together with human RIG 20 IU/kg.

It is of interest to note that 37 of 38 travellers who had received pre-exposure rabies vaccination, irrespective of the route, showed seroprotective levels of rabies antibody (>0.5 IU/mL) after 5 years (Katmandu, 2006).

Note the definition of an anamnestic response: renewed rapid production of an antibody on the second (or subsequent) encounter with the same antigen.

52. C. It is important to give as much of the RIG possible in and around the wound. Give the rest IM, never IV. RIG is important, even a year after the incident, because rabies can have a long incubation period. Equine RIG is more widely available than human RIG.

53. B. Children are much more likely to approach and pet animals than adults. In Nepal monkeys still account for less than half of the rabies exposure in tourists. Canine rabies still predominates in Thailand. A rabid animal may appear quiet and docile during the phase of CNS depression and still be capable of transmitting the disease. Fatal imported rabies was recorded in the UK from dog bites in 2005 (Goa) and in 2009 (South Africa). Bat-transmitted rabies is notorious in Texas. European bat lyssavirus type 2 is endemic in bat populations in countries otherwise considered free from rabies, e.g. the UK.

54. D. At least seven people have died from rabies following transplants from donors who had recently been bitten by rabid dogs or bats. PreEP alone does not prevent rabies. PreEP merely primes the immune system to respond vigorously to PoEP without the need for RIG. Some immunity for 1 year has been found after two ID doses of vaccine at different sites (both deltoids) given at one visit a week before departure. Almost half of the worldwide deaths from rabies occur in children (bites on hands, face, or neck).

Unique in the literature is the report of a 15-year-old girl who survived bat rabies despite receiving neither PoEP nor RIG. There is an anecdotal report of rabies having been transmitted by the bite of a rabid mother to her son in Ethiopia (personal case).

55. C. Routine pneumococcal vaccines for adults contain a mixture of capsular polysaccharides from 23 of the most common and most invasive pneumococci.

Invasive pneumococcal disease includes meningitis, pneumonia, and general sepsis. Non-invasive types cause sinusitis, otitis media, and broncitis.

56. C. The vaccine gives a very poor antibody response in those under 2 years of age. A seven-valent conjugate vaccine CRM197, e.g. Prenvar®, is given to children 6 weeks to 5 years old. Nonetheless the polyvalent non-conjugated vaccine is useful for those with a transplant history, asplenia, chronic illness, the elderly, and anyone at high risk from pneumococcal infections because of their work, e.g. nurses and school teachers. It is also recommended for selected groups, e.g. those with haemoglobinopathies, the immunocompromised, or those with potential CSF leaks, e.g. ventriculo-atrial shunts or cochlear implants. The protection after a single dose lasts about 5 years. Antibody response is established 3 weeks after vaccination.

57. B. Although pneumococci are the most common cause of pneumonia there is no evidence that vaccinaton reduces the risk in travellers. However, it is routinely given to healthy adults at 65 years of age and over, whether or not they travel overseas. There is no blanket recommendation for giving it to any of the other groups listed, although individuals within these groups may require the vaccine. Pneumococci are responsible for more deaths than any other bacteria for which a vaccine exists. CDC suggest that, because of a poor response to repeated doses, those over 65 years of age should not be re-vaccinated if they were 65 years old at time of their last vaccination.

58. D. Influenza virus is grown on chick eggs and therefore is contraindicated if the recipient is known to have definite egg allergy. The vaccine must not be frozen. It contains sub-particles of two or all three influenza types. This applies whether the vaccine is surface antigen, virosomal, or split virion.

59. C. Breast-feeding is NOT a contraindication to receiving the influenza vaccine.

The influenza season is November to March in northern parts and April to September south of the equator. It is present in all seasons in the tropics. Vaccine contains thiomersal preservative (approximately 50 % ethylmercury) and it will take some time before mercury-free vaccine is widely available. The vaccine does not contain penicillin. The success of the vaccine you give depends largely on matching the antigen of the vaccine strains administered with the current circulating influenza strains. There may be a north–south mismatch in this respect. Guidelines for protection are issued by WHO in February for the northern hemisphere and in October for the southern hemisphere.

60. C. Combination of influenza vaccine with an adjuvant improves immunogenicity but also increases the frequency of post-immunization reactions. Amantidine and its derivatives are used widely as influenza prophylactics but are far inferior to the vaccine. The effectiveness of the vaccine decreases in the elderly, who need it more than younger people. Young people on long-term aspirin therapy are at increased risk of getting Reyes syndrome after influenza and therefore should be vaccinated. Links between swine flu vaccine and narcolepsy have not been established (2012).

61. B. Tick-borne encephalitis is transmitted by ticks to well over 100 species of wild and domestic animals (sheep, goats, dogs, cattle) and humans. Unlike Lyme disease, doxycycline is ineffective and there is no specific treatment. Tick-borne encephalitis is currently found only in Eurasia. Tick-borne encephalitis is a flavivirus, like yellow fever, dengue fever, and Japanese encephalitis.

62. A. Tick-borne encephalitis vaccine is a suspension of purified formaldehyde-inactivated tick-borne encephalitis virus propagated on chick embryo cells. Usually three doses are given (0, 4–12 weeks, and booster at 1 year). This gives substantial protection against all tick-borne encephalitis strains in Europe and Asia. One should try to give the second dose at least 2 weeks before departure to high-risk areas, although even one dose can result in protective antibody levels. An accelerated vaccination schedule (day 0, 7, and 21) has proved efficacious. A junior preparation is available from 1 year up to the 16th birthday.

63. C. The danger of meningitis is greatest in the dry season. The African 'meningitis belt' extends from the Bight of Benin to Somalia but outbreaks have also been reported recently from Angola, Rwanda, Tanzania, and the Congo. Protection in adults starts after 10 days and lasts about 2–3 years whether the vaccine is conjugated or not. Polysaccharide vaccines are poorly immunogenic in infants. Like other conjugate vaccines, the quadrivalent conjugate ACYW-135 (Menveo®,MCV4®, Menactra®) and the monovalent C conjugate vaccine have good immunogenicity in infants, and have been approved in the USA for those between 9 months and 55 years (Advisory Committee on Immunization Practice, 2010).

Since *N. meningitidis* is found in the nasal passages of almost 25% of adolescents only conjugate vaccine should be given to this group.

64. C. There was a serious outbreak of W-135 meningitis in Burkina Faso in 2002 and W-135 is reported from many places in Africa now. Serotype A is declining somewhat. The glycoconjugate vaccine is expensive but affords better protection than the polysaccharide one. The timing of boosters is not yet settled (2012). No cross-protection is afforded against other meningitis serotypes.

65. B. The incidence of hepatitis A has declined tenfold in developing countries in recent times, although there are still many high-risk places where non-immunized people eat and drink recklessly.

Hepatitis A has a higher incidence in travellers than legionella but a lower incidence than influenza, malaria, animal bites, dengue fever, PPD conversion, and TD. Some authorities suggest the risk of acquiring hepatitis A is 3/1000/month in non-immunized travellers. In very chaotic situations, e.g. refugee camps, the risk is even higher. Note that staying in a five-star hotel does NOT eliminate the risk of getting hepatitis A.

The risk of acquiring heptitis A is particularly high if you eat raw seafood or seafood in which the core temperature does not exceed 70°C (very common) even in developed countries, e.g. in Puglia, Italy.

66. C. Inactivated vaccine is used widely. It is considered safe in lactation but, because of lack of data, should be avoided in pregnancy unless deemed essential (CDC, 2011). A live attenuated vaccine is manufactured in China but is not in general use elsewhere.

67. A. If allergy to aluminium is present then it is advisable to switch from a regular hepatis A vaccine to Epaxil™ (SSI, Berna) which only uses formaldehyde and thiomersal as preservatives. VAQTA™ (Merck) is free of preservatives (see manufacturer's leaflet).

68. A. About 80% of those vaccinated have protective levels of anti-HAV after 2 weeks (>33 mIU/ml) and one expects >90% protection after 4 weeks. While a booster at 6 months is recommended it is accepted now that a booster is effective if given up to 5 years later. A booster dose probably covers the patient for life. Junior preparations of Havrix and Vaqta are available for those <16 years of age. Note that either post-exposure vaccination or anti-HAV immunoglobulin can be given after probable exposure.

69. B. Hepatitis B vaccine gives a less than expected response in smokers, older people, the immunocompromised, and those with impaired renal function. It will have a predictable response in those on hemodialysis unless they are immunocompromised. Athleticism *per se* is not an issue. Simultaneous administration of HBV Ig will not impair the response to the vaccine if given at a different site.

70. C. Obesity, male gender, old age, a history of smoking, and pre-existing serious medical conditions can all reduce immunogenicity.

71. D. Avoid giving hepatitis B vaccine to a pregnant or breast-feeding mother unless there is an overriding imperative. So far there are no studies to confirm or refute any ill-effects on the foetus or on the breast-fed infant. The immunocompromised require larger doses of non-live vaccines than normal in order to mount a satisfactory response. Children as young as 1 or 2 years can receive a reduced dose as can neonates, especially those born to mothers who are HBV carriers. A paediatric suspension is available. Hepatitis B vaccine can be given to elderly travellers, although they often show a poor immunogenic response. Patients with impaired renal function, including those on haemodialysis, have a reduced immune response to hepatitis B vaccine and need double doses of the vaccine given in the normal timeframe.

72. B. Hepatitis B vaccine is currently used in the national immunization programmes of over 150 countries. Over 1000 million doses of the vaccine have been used. The suggestion of Dr Miguel Hernan et al. in 2004 that immunization against hepatitis B is associated with a threefold increase in the incidence of MS 'within 3 years following vaccination' has been refuted. Reports of a causal link with CFS (syn. post viral fatigue syndrome), SIDS, Parkinson's disease, and a variety of demyelinating diseases have also been discredited. Hepatitis B vaccine is probably one of the safest vaccines in use. It is indicated for travel to places where carriage rates are above 2% or when the traveller is likely to engage in activities which place them at risk of infection.

73. C. Hepatitis B can be a very severe disease in those who already have hepatitis C and immunization against HBV is strongly recommended. The vaccine contains recombinant adsorbed HbsAg (HBV surface antigen). It is given in a dose of 20 μg to those over 15 years of age. A junior preparation is given to younger patients.

Today's vaccines are made from recombinant HBsAg grown in yeast. They are thiomersal free.

74. B. In the clinical disease only anti-HBs (that is antibody against the HBV surface antigen) leads to recovery. Most consider that protection is present when anti HBsAg levels of >10 IU/ml are found, although some have set a limit of 100 IU/ml. HBc refers to the core antigen, HBe to the antigen that encapsulates the viral DNA, the infective part of the virus.

75. D. Seroprotective levels of anti-HBV keep rising in most vaccinees, so that about 90% of recipients are protected after a year. Levels after a month vary widely, but rarely reach 10 IU/ml (seroprotection). If a booster is given then you may expect close to >90% seroprotection. A similar situation pertains to combined hepatitis A and B vaccine. Approximately 5–10% of healthy individuals fail to achieve an adequate antibody response whatever schedule is used.

76. A. Many believe that after a successful primary series of hepatitis B vaccine one is protected for life. However, while infants and children have a non-responder rate of <5% this rises to over 10% in adults.

In non-responders, administration of one or two more doses or concomitant administration of doses in right and left deltoids on one or two occasions can raise the response rate. A third-generation hepatitis B vaccine is in the pipeline.

77. D. A three-dose schedule is required for a seroprotective response, that is, >33 IU/ml anti-HAV and >10 IU/ml anti-HBs antibody. Pooled data from six studies shows that the combined vaccine gives just as good immunity as the monodose vaccines.Combined A and B vaccines do not give significantly more local reactions than their separate components. Boostering specifically for either type with the combined vaccine is not always effective. Refer to the manufacturer's leaflet re boostering usage.

78. C. HBV Ig gives short-term protection for those at very 'high risk'. Thus it can be given to non-responders who will be involved in invasive surgical procedures in highly endemic areas. It can be used in post-exposure treatment, although a rapid schedule of active vaccination is more appropriate. As a rule avoid blood products as much as possible.

79. A. Jane Zuckerman et al. found that the increase in geometric mean antibody titre after a standard dose of Avaxim (160GMB U^3) was significantly greater than that following Havrix (1440 units/ml). Pain at the injection site was also significantly more common after Havrix. In all other respects, both preparations were safe and equally well tolerated. In Beeching's study (2004) both vaccines induced high levels of protective antibodies and neither was associated with any serious adverse effects. Current evidence suggests that other vaccines against hepatitis A, e.g. Epaxal® and Vaqta®, are interchangeable with Havrix and Avaxim. Seroprotective levels, that is, a titre >10 mIU/l, are achieved by all these vaccines.

A dose of 0.5 ml of Epaxal contains 24 IU of inactivated HAV adsorbed on adjuvant virosomes, which are purified influenza virus surface antigens. Epaxal is aluminium free.

A second dose of any of the above vaccines provides at least 30 years of cover. Pediatric preparations are available for hepatitis A vaccines.

80. D. Overbosch et al. (2005) showed that a combined vaccine (Viatim™) was as tolerable, immunogenic, and safe as the individual vaccines. In the case of the first combined vaccine (Hepatyrix™), Beran et al. (2000) showed that >95% of the recipients became positive for anti-Vi antibodies and >86% positive for anti-HAV antibodies after 14 days. Beeching et al. (2004) confirmed this and also showed that the typhoid responses were higher and the hepatitis A responses more rapid after Viatim™. Nonetheless they also showed that Viatim™ elicited more local responses than Hepatyrix™ (82.7% versus 53.1%).

81. C. Modern injectable capsular polysaccharide typhoid vaccine (ViCPS) comprises a non-live antigen that retains its potency even if kept for a week at 25°C and for more than a day at 37°C. This is important to know if a traveller carries the vaccine overseas. The vaccine only protects against *S. typhi* (CDC, 2012). Do not give to children <2 years old.

82. C. One should wait until the patient is afebrile before giving parenteral typhoid vaccine. The other options are not relevant.

83. A. Although values vary considerably, protection falls from a high of around >80% in 3 months to about 50% in 3 years.

84. D. Oral typhoid vaccine is a live attenuated vaccine containing 2×10^9 *S. typhi* Ty21a organisms per capsule. The capsules must be refrigerated and taken on an empty stomach 1 hour before a meal.

85. A. Protection is present after a week, is usually about 50% after 3 years, and, exceptionally, as high as 67% after 7 years. A booster is recommended every 3 years for ViCPS and every 6 years for Ty21a. Do not break the enteric-coated capsules because stomach acidity may reduce vaccine efficacy despite buffer in the capsule.

Capsules should be kept at 1–5°C and not used if outside this range for 48 hours. Capsules are taken with a liquid no warmer than 37°C, approximately 1 hour before a meal. The US schedule is superior to the three-dose schedule used in Europe.

Do not give this vaccine to children under 6 years of age.

86. C. It is important to complete the schedule correctly whether you use a three- or four-dose regime. Extending the periods between dosing reduces the efficacy of the series. Since it is a live vaccine it should not be given to immunocompromised individuals or in pregnancy. Concomitant antibiotics or diarrhoea impair efficacy but normal eating does not. *S. typhi* is not found in the stools of vacinees. Separate the taking of mefloquine or chloroquin by 8 hours.

87. A. Falling levels of anti-HAV in donor plasma have meant that nowadays the efficacy of HIG in protecting against HAV is vastly reduced. Most countries no longer supply HIG for this purpose. Modern HIG is screened for HCV, HIV, and many other infectious agents.

88. D. Varicella vaccine is a live attenuated vaccine. Plague vaccine is an inactivated whole-cell vaccine. A vaccine against Lyme disease has been developed in the Czech Republic (2008). The inactivated US vaccine has been off the market for some years, apparently because of cost issues.

Anthrax vaccine is an inactivated vaccine produced from culture filtrates of an avirulent, non-encapsulated B anthracis and is given in three doses. Anthrax vaccine is currently on the restricted list. The vaccine contains aluminium.

89. C. Rabies vaccine stimulates memory T-cells and thus a booster injection dose gives added stimulus to primed T-cells. Polysaccharide vaccines such as *S. typhi* Vi, quadrivalent meningococcal vaccine or Pneumovax® only involve B-cells and do not involve T-cells (memory cells). Thus there is no question of 'boostering' the initial immunity with a subsequent dose. Their protective effect is essentially finished after a certain length of time and one must begin all over again. Conjugate vaccines, where there is a protein adjunct, involve long-term immunity.

90. D. Plague vaccine is a suspension of inactivated *P. pestis* organisms. Apart from a few military personnel who got the plague in Vietnam there have been few studies on the efficacy of the vaccine. At best it may only give 50–60% protection after three injections over 6 months. While it may be somewhat effective against rat-flea transmitted disease it appears unlikely to protect against the aerosol-transmitted variety (pneumonic plague). The vaccine should not be given to children <11 years old.

Plague is an infection of wild rodents and is transmitted by rat fleas. The vaccine is very occasionally advised for those going to be in very close contact with rodents in infected areas. The black rat is renowned for carrying fleas on ships.

Diagnosed early, plague is readily curable using tetracycline or chloramphenicol.

Risk areas include Africa (sub-Saharan Africa), the Americas (Western USA, Bolivia, Brazil, Ecuador, Peru), and Asia (Vietnam, near Caspian sea).

Apart from selected military and laboratory personnel, the vaccine may also be indicated for anyone who has regular conact with rodents in plague endemic locations.

91. B. Zoster vaccine (Zostvax®) was licensed in the USA in 2006 and is very effective in preventing shingles and post-herpetic neuralgia, which typically affect older people as well as those under stress. Zoster vaccine is a live vaccine and given as a single dose. Unfortunately it is expensive. This man fits both criteria and is unlikely to have access to this vaccine in Angola. Pertussis infections account for 40% of chronic cough in adults and the vaccine is being used more and more in travel clinics although it has not entered the mainstream of travel vaccines yet.

Recall that sero-immunity to pertussis from childhood vaccination only lasts 10 years.

Varicella vaccine is very effective against chicken pox but gives little protection against shingles. One might consider anthrax protection for an agricultural worker, but no cases have been reported from Angola in recent times. It is interesting to note that four cases of polio were confirmed in Angola in 2011.

PRE-TRAVEL CONSULTATION

QUESTIONS

The importance of a comprehensive pre-travel consultation cannot be overemphasized. Each clinic should have a detailed questionnaire that the traveller can fill out while waiting. Details of past history, a list of past vaccinations, known allergies, current medications, the planned itinerary, the length of stay, the time of year, and proposed activities are all important as well as age, sex, pregnancy, medical travel insurance, and contact numbers.

Such a review is extremely helpful and cuts down on the time required when the traveller is admitted to see you.

General

1. **The most important segment of the pre-travel consultation is**
   A. Administration of vaccines
   B. Giving antimalarial chemoprophylaxis when travelling to a malaria endemic country
   C. Giving advice about personal protection against possible illness
   D. Explaining cultural differences

2. **Which do you consider the most important information document that a traveller should carry?**
   A. A list of known allergies
   B. International driving license (if planning to drive)
   C. Blood type and group
   D. Travel insurance card

3. **Which of the following is the most important advice to give the traveller?**
   A. Carry money on your person
   B. Take a small amount of cash and only one credit card
   C. Carry a photocopy of your passport
   D. Have a contact telephone number for your country's embassy at your destination

4. **When a traveller is on an oral contraceptive (OC)**
   A. She should be sure to take her OC at the same time each day irrespective of the number of time zones crossed
   B. She can be assured that there is no increased risk of venous thrombosis
   C. She should use an alternative method of contraception for the first 2–3 weeks while on doxycycline
   D. Absorption of her OC is decreased if she gets diarrhoea

5. **Fitness to travel, where there is a known cardiac disease, is primarily the responsibility of the**
   A. Traveller
   B. Cardiologist
   C. Travel clinic nurse or doctor
   D. Airline, provided advance warning is given

6. **Which of the following do you consider the best source of information concerning travel health risks in a particular country?**
   A. Local health officials in that country
   B. TV health programmes/newspapers
   C. The embassy of the country in question
   D. The internet, e.g. CDC, WHO, Travax

7. **Medical facilities abroad**
   A. Can be relied on for the diagnosis of local endemic diseases
   B. Are best identified via embassy or consular staff in the host country
   C. Should be given in a list to all travellers
   D. Need to be discussed with all intending travellers

Specific

1. **A patient had a small spontaneous pneumothorax 3 weeks ago. He plans to fly across the Atlantic. What should you say to him?**
   A. Postpone the flight for 6 weeks
   B. Postpone the flight for 6 months
   C. Request oxygen from the airline if he flies within 1 year
   D. Fly any time provided he can walk 50 m on the flat without any discomfort

2. **Which of these is the most important single piece of advice for preventing diarrhoea in wilderness backpackers?**
   A. Carry a fluoroquinolone antibiotic
   B. Carry a quantity of oral rehydration solution
   C. Only drink surface water in pristine areas
   D. Hand wash after urination

3. **Which of these is the most important/best prophylaxis for short-term visitors to a malaria endemic area?**
   A. Appropriate chemoprophylaxis
   B. Standby emergency standby treatment (SBET)
   C. Personal protective measures
   D. Air conditioning

4. **You can assure patients that there is no schistosomiasis in**
   A. Venezuela
   B. Vietnam
   C. Dominica
   D. India

5. **When the new vaccine against Lyme disease (borreliosis) becomes available one should consider giving it to all hill walkers between 15 and 70 years old who plan treks in**
   A. Wooded areas of New Jersey in summer
   B. The Bavarian Alps in September
   C. The Swiss Alps in August
   D. Any of these locations

6. **A nurse comes to your clinic and says she 'got a course of hepatitis B injections about 7 years ago' but produces no documentary evidence. She plans to do voluntary work in a clinic in South Africa. Would you**
   A. Assume she is protected against hepatitis B
   B. Test her blood for hepatitis B surface *antigen* levels and then decide what to do
   C. Test her blood for hepatitis B surface *antibody* and then decide what to do
   D. Give her hepatitis B vaccine at this visit

7. **A prospective traveller tells you that he has heard that immunization against hepatitis B protects against some other type of hepatitis. You tell him that hepatitis B immunization only protects against**
   A. Hepatitis B
   B. Hepatitis B and hepatitis C
   C. Hepatitis B and hepatitis D
   D. Hepatitis B and hepatitis E

8. **Which of the following blood findings is used to show protection against future hepatitis B infection and indicate that the person is a non-carrier of the disease?**
   A. Hepatitis B surface antibody (anti-HBs)
   B. Hepatitis B surface antigen (HBsAg)
   C. Hepatitis B e-antigen (HBeAg)
   D. Anti-hepatitis B core antigen (anti-HBcAg)

9. **A traveller going for the first time alone to Nairobi should be warned to**
   A. Use only a clearly licensed taxi at the airport
   B. Book hotel reservations in advance for the first night
   C. Make sure that he has his entry tax in hard currency
   D. Make sure he is taking his antimalarial tablets

10. **Would you believe a prospective traveller to East Africa who tells you**
   A. Tsetse flies only bite at night
   B. Red wine with food kills enteropathogens
   C. Still water in a sealed bottle is safe to drink
   D. 'Mosquitoes love me'

11. **What is the *lowest temperature* food must reach for 1 minute in order to destroy most important enteropathogens?**
   A. 45°C
   B. 65°C
   C. 85°C
   D. 100°C

12. **Solid organ transplant recipients**
   A. Should avoid live vaccines, e.g. yellow fever
   B. Have an increased risk of graft rejection after vaccination
   C. Can be considered functionally asplenic
   D. Will fail to produce a full response to most vaccines until at least 6 months have elapsed since their last dose of immunosuppressive agents such as cyclosporine, steroids, methotrexate, or azathioprine

13. **Travellers taking steroids**
   A. Have virtually no antibody response to live vaccines
   B. Have a normal antibody response to inactivated vaccines
   C. Have a significantly increased risk of opportunistic infections
   D. Have the same immune status for a given dose of any steroid irrespective of how it is delivered

14. **A 30-year-old male traveller plans to travel to Bangkok on 2 August for 4 weeks. He has had no previous travel vaccines. You see him on 29 July. Which is the most appropriate *single vaccine* you would recommend from the list below?**
   A. Hepatitis A
   B. Typhoid
   C. Hepatitis B
   D. Diphtheria/tetanus

15. **A 30-year-old male plans to hike in the Atlas Mountains in Morocco, leaving on 2 August. He sees you on 29 July. Which of the following is he most likely to contract?**
    A. Polio
    B. Diphtheria/tetanus
    C. Hepatitis A
    D. Tick-borne encephalitis

16. **A 40-year-old man is going to work for the local power company in Uzbekistan. Apart from the usual vaccines, which of the following do you consider most appropriate?**
    A. Anthrax
    B. Plague
    C. Japanese encephalitis vaccine
    D. Rabies

17. **A business man is travelling to Pakistan and plans to stay in a village after his business is done in Karachi. With regards to malaria should you**
    A. Assure him that Karachi is malaria free
    B. Suggest he take doxycycline or atovaquone/proguanil or mefloquine as a malarial prophylactic
    C. Suggest he take chloroquin and proguanil
    D. Suggest he bring standby emergency treatment

18. **Which is the best way to avoid schistosomiasis?**
    A. Apply a solution of 50% DEET (diethyltoluamide) to the skin immediately after exposure
    B. Have an immediate vigorous rub down with a towel after exposure
    C. Only swim in deep water (>2 m)
    D. Only swim in chlorinated swimming pools

General

1. C. Time spent in clearly explaining about accidental injury, insect bites, food and water hazards, exessive exposure to the sun and any dangers inherent in special activities, e.g. leptospirosis in water sports, rabies in cave explorers, is the most important segment of any pre-travel consultation. You must be sure that the patient fully understands such dangers and promises to take personal protective measures against them.

2. A. If one is truly allergic to a particular item then it is essential that this be made known or be readily accessible to others, irrespective of location. Every country has its own regulations re driving permits and this should be checked in advance. Should a blood transfusion be absolutely necessary to save life, then even poorly equipped hospitals can do typing and cross-matching. Travel insurance information should be carried or at least readily authenticated by phone, fax, or email.

3. C. Most travellers are well aware of the best way to take money, but few will photostat important documents, in particular their passport, which it is vital to have in case of loss or theft or difficulties with the local authorities. A simple way is to email the relevant page to your own phone. Note too that many places have no facilities to cash cheques or have either suspect or no ATM machines.

Travellers should be advised never change money unofficially. Travellers have been caught and jailed when duped by local police 'plants'. Neither should they trust the 'safes' in hotel bedrooms, irrespective of the hotel's grading. Telephones frequently do not work and if help is needed then any friendly embassy will put a traveller in touch with their own one.

4. D. Be sure to inform women that diarrhoea can interfere with the absorption of OCs. Always take an OC so that there is 24-hour cover irrespective of number of time zones crossed.

The risk of venous thrombosis is always increased in those on OCs and such individuals are more likely to develop an air-travel-related DVT than others.

Nowadays it is understood that doxycycline does not reduce the contraceptive action of oestrogen-containing OCs.

5. C. If there is any doubt about the fitness of an individual to travel then is the duty of the travel clinic to consult with the traveller's cardiologist. It is not the airline's responsibility nor is it the patient's, although he or she can take responsibility by signing a witnessed document to that effect.

6. D. In general, internet sources, such as WHO, CDC, Travax and the International Society of Travel Medicine, are the most reliable.

Newspapers and TV programmes are notoriously sensational and inaccurate, while embassies paint an overly ' healthy' picture of their countries.

Local health officials in some countries are unreliable sources of information.

7. D. The location, the competence, and the payment for medical facilities abroad should be discussed with all travellers, especially those who are pregnant, elderly, or have any pre-exisitng illness. In addition, these travellers should have the telephone number of the nearest embassy, have a printed list and an adequate supply of medications, have the email address of their home doctor, and check that their insurance will cover all medical expenses.

Many facilities overseas are excellent; many are not. The over-diagnosis of malaria in travellers in malaria-endemic countries is a case in point.

Contact numbers such as that for the International Association for Medical Assistance to Travellers (IAMAT) should be available in your clinic. See chapter 13.

Specific

1. A. Most agree that an air trip should be postponed for at least 6 weeks after a pneumothorax. Individual physicians may opt to be even more cautious, remembering that there is a 50% chance of recurrence within a year of getting a first pneumothorax.

2. D. The incidence of diarrhoea is least in backpackers who hand wash after urination. Hand sanitizers should also be used. Other advice to prevent diarrhoea includes washing post-defecation, cleaning cooking utensils in hot soapy water using the three-bowl washing routine, disinfecting all drinking water, and taking probiotics and multivitamin tablets. See chapter 9.

3. C. One cannot get malaria if one is not bitten. Correct and regular protective measures should be a priority. This includes repellents, impregnated nets, screening of windows, insecticide sprays, and air-conditioning with proper mesh filters on the inlet orifices. Appropriate chemoprophylaxis implies taking the correct anti-malarial conscientiously and in accordance with instructions, e.g. same time of day and mostly with food.

SBET is being adopted widely but remember that SBET is only to be used when medical help is more than 24 hours away and when, in a risk area, symptoms and signs strongly suggest malaria, e.g. sudden onset of high fever, rigors, and headache. See chapter 14.

4. D. Schistosomiasis does not occur in India. It is largely confined to Venezuela and Brazil in South America. It has been eliminated from the Caribbean with the exception of pockets of *S. mansoni* in St Lucia and the Dominican Republic. *S. mekongi* is found in the Mekong delta of Vietnam.

5. D. There are three known species of Borrelia. Only one species is known to exist in the USA, the others are found in Europe and Asia. The original vaccine, Lymerix, was only effective against the US strain. It was made from killed borrelia and was about 75% effective against the clinical disease.

The bioengineered Czech vaccine (targeted against borrelia surface proteins) appears to be effective against all species of borrelia. It should be in use by 2015.

6. C. You cannot be sure, even with a nurse, that she got the full course of primary injections against hepatitis B. The wisest thing to do is to test her blood for hepatitis B surface antibody in order to establish her immune status. Anyone going to an area where the hepatitis B carriage rate is >2% should be protected.

7. C. Immunization against HBV will protect against HDV. Hepatitis D is caused by a defective RNA virus that can only replicate in the presence of hepatitis B.

8. A. Anti-HBs indicates past exposure to HBV, including past immunization and immunity to the disease. The virus is no longer present and the person cannot transmit HBV.

HBsAG is found in active disease and, although it disappears during recovery, it may reappear in chronic disease, especially in children and in the immunocompromised. HBsAG is also called the Australian antigen because it was discovered in an Australian aborigine by Baruch Blumberg, an American.

HBeAG is only found in blood when the actual virus is present and is used as a marker of infectivity (carrier state).

Anti-HBcAg is an antibody to the HBV core antigen and is usually found in carriers. It indicates either present or past HBV infection.

People who have occult HBV in the liver with a very low viraemia are infective and are called 'carriers'. They may feel quite well themselves or progress to overt liver damage or liver cancer.

9. A. There have been several unhappy incidents involving unlicensed taxis in Nairobi, as in other cities. If it is not possible to be met, then it is wise to seek advice from the airport tourist office about transport and hotels. Refuse any offers of a ride from unauthorized people. It is convenient but not essential to have booked one's first night. There is no need to take malaria chemoprophylaxis in Nairobi itself.

10. D. Some people are more attractive to mosquitoes by virtue of sex, skin colour, hormonal status, and their eccrine and apocrine secretions. Tsetse flies bite at any time and, while red wine kills some enteropathogens in vitro, there is no substantial evidence that it kills enteropathogens when taken with a meal. Sealed carbonated bottle water is probably safe, apparently sealed still water may not be. Remember the utensil you are drinking from may not be clean.

11. B. Important enteropathogens are destroyed if brought to just over 60°C. Unfortunately not all parts of the cooked meal may have reached this temperature. Also bear in mind that some non-food or non-water-borne enteric pathogens, e.g. clostridial spores, can survive up to 100°C for many minutes. Remember too that it may be the condiment, sauce, dressing, or surrounding side dishes that carry the pathogen. In many restaurants, fish are kept alive in tanks filled with polluted water. This poses its own risks. Epidemics of cholera and hepatitis have occurred in highly respectable areas of Hong Kong because of this.

12. A. A yellow fever waiver should be given to all such patients going to yellow fever endemic areas. Those who have had allogenic bone marrow transplant for blood disease can be considered functionally asplenic but not those with solid organ transplants, e.g. kidney and liver. Immunosuppression can last for 3 months after taking any of the drugs mentioned in the question.

13. C. Even 20 mg of prednisone a day can lead to an increased risk of opportunistic infection. Steroids reduce the immune response to all vaccines, yet surprisingly those on steroids have a good response to influenza vaccine. When steroids are injected into a closed space (joint/bursa) systemic absorption is slowed and thus the patient is effectively on a lower dose of the drug. Live vaccines are contraindicated if the subject is on steroids.

14. A. Hepatitis A is the most common infection acquired by travellers worldwide. In general terms it occurs 1–3/1000 non-immunized persons per week of travel. The vaccine is safe and efficient, and can be given at the last minute.

15. C. Hepatitis A.

16. D. Ubzekistan is classified as a high-risk country for rabies. Japanese encephalitis vaccine conjugate vaccine should also be considered if spending >4 months in a rural area. Infected culex mosquitoes that transmit Japanese encephalitis are common. Tick-bourne encephalitis, TB, polio, and very rarely anthrax and plague are also hazards.

17. B. Both *P. vivax* and *P. falciparum* are endemic in Pakistan below 2000 m. Outbreaks have been reported from many areas, including Karachi, where it has been shown that resistance to chloroquin varies from 16% to 62%. July to November are the worst months but recently outbreaks have occurred in April and May, and all year long in the Sindh Province.The anopheles mosquito breeds in clear water and breeding places are increasing in the expanding cities of Pakistan, India, and Bangladesh due to the number of unattended pools of water engendered by construction sites. Some authorities, especially in mainland Europe, recommend SBET. For SBET to be a good choice the patient must be instructed properly about its use and its limitations.

18. A. There are several reports showing that even modest concentrations of DEET applied to the skin immediately after bathing can prevent schistosomiasis. Cercariae take about 5–15 minutes to penetrate the skin and it is during this stage that they are vulnerable to DEET.

A report on Peace Corps Volunteers shows that only one in 11 of those who rubbed down well after swimming in Lake Malawi contracted the disease so this practice should not be disregarded. However, swimming in deep water, in fast-flowing water, or in luxury swimming pools has not prevented cercariae penetrating the skin. Always warn against swimming in endemic areas.

Dermatosis is one of the top four problems that affect travellers. Sunburn is high on the list, especially, but not exclusively, in those who travel to sun resorts. Occasionally medication-related photosensitivity dermatitis occurs and travellers should be warned to immediately stop taking the suspected allergen when this occurs. For example, should photosensitivity occur when taking doxycycline, a failure to stop the drug immediately together with persistent exposure to the sun can result in a serious exfoliative dermatitis that may need hospitalization. Apart from those dermatoses that are found in temperate climates, there are a number of tropical and parasitic-related skin conditions with which the travel medicine practitioner should be familiar.

Skin and sun

1. **Regarding ultraviolet (UV) sun rays, UVA and UVB**
   A. UVA is more likely to cause sunburn than UVB
   B. UVA and UVB are equally damaging to the skin
   C. During midday, the amount of UVB reaching the skin is 100 times greater than the amount of UVA
   D. People over 65 are more likely to develop solar keratosis when exposed to sunlight

2. **Which of the following is good advice regarding sun blockers and UV sunlight?**
   A. Reapply sun blocker after a minimum of 8 hours
   B. The effects of UV on the skin wear off in 4 weeks
   C. Physical blockers are often allergenic
   D. Chemical blockers absorb light

3. **Which of the following is true concerning sun blockers?**
   A. The skin protection factor (SPF) of a preparation is determined by the time it takes erythema to appear after exposure to sunlight
   B. Do not use SPF > 10 on a 4-month-old baby
   C. An SPF of at least 60 should be applied to fair-skinned adults who sunbathe
   D. Physical blockers only filter out UVA

4. **Which of the following are common beliefs about sun blockers?**
    A. Some preparations are waterproof
    B. Some preparations can facilitate the development of skin cancer
    C. Apply immediately before exposure for best effects
    D. They are most useful when mixed with insect repellents

Insect repellents

1. **Which of the following is true regarding DEET's protection?**
    A. DEET is more protective against *Anopheles* spp. than against *Culex* spp.
    B. DEET is more protective against *Anopheles* spp. than against *Aedes* spp.
    C. DEET gives excellent protection against insects when impregnated on a wristband
    D. DEET is very useful in protecting against arthropods when applied to cotton or nylon jackets

2. **DEET**
    A. Affects the odour sensors of mosquitoes
    B. Is a 'knockdown' insect repellent
    C. Effectiveness increases in a linear fashion until its concentration exceeds 50%
    D. Effectiveness is reduced if applied under a chemical sunblock cream

3. **Permethrin is**
    A. A synthetic repellent related to DEET
    B. Activated by our skin oils
    C. Active for 6 months once applied
    D. Far superior to DEET in repelling ticks

4. **Icaridin (picaridin, KBR3032) is**
    A. Likely to damage plastic, e.g. watch straps
    B. Comparable to DEET in similar concentrations
    C. Contraindicated in children under 6 years old
    D. Ineffective against *An. gambiae*

5. **Which of these repellents is superior to the others?**
    A. Lemon eucalyptus oil
    B. Garlic
    C. Citronella
    D. Oral vitamin B

Skin and sun

1. D. Older people are far more likely to develop solar keratoses than others. UVB is more likely to cause sunburn, keratoses, skin cancer, and skin ageing than UVA. UVB (290–320 nm) has a shorter wavelength than UVA (320–400 nm) and so doea not penetrate the skin as deeply. However, at midday, UVA radiation pierces the skin more deeply than UVB because its strength at this time is 10 times more intense than that of UVB. Thus UVA becomes a greater threat—including for skin cancer—at a time when many travellers are sunbathing or taking part in activities such as climbing or skiing. Note that UV light is ultimately more damaging to the skin of children than to any other age group.

2. D. Chemical blockers, e.g. *para*-aminobenzoic acid (PABA), camphor derivative, and benzophenones, absorb light. Physical ones, e.g. zinc oxide and titanium dioxide, reflect, scatter, and absorb light. One should reapply a sunscreen after 3–6 hours. Chemical blockers are often allergenic and may cause photosensitization.

3. A. SPF is the ratio of the time needed to produce minimal erythema on factor-treated skin to the time taken to produce the same erythema on uncovered skin.

An SPF of 15 is safe for children <6 months old. Ideally small children should not be exposed to direct sunlight without protection, e.g. a sun shade or hat.

An SPF of at least 30 is recommended for fair-skinned adults but do not forget that UVB can cause sunburn in dark-skinned people too. Physical blockers may be unsightly but are the best. They are rarely allergenic and can completely block both UVA and UVB.

4. B. A chemical blocker that is effective in preventing sunburn (UVB) may not be nearly as effective in blocking UVA. Thus the user may lie in the sun for long periods during which excess UVA penetrates the skin and initiates loss of elastic tissue, skin sagging, wrinkles, skin pigmentation, and even cancer. No preparation is completely waterproof. This is especially important when applying protective creams and sprays to children who are in and out of swimming pools. Blockers should be applied 10–30 minutes before exposure to the sun and any mixture with insect repellents is best avoided.

Insect repellents

1. D. Application of DEET to wide-mesh cotton/nylon gives good protection against mosquitoes and biting flies. Some hold that it is worth applying it to wristbands. Field studies have shown that

DEET gives more protection against biting *Culex* spp., *Aedes* spp., *Mansonia* spp., and *Verallina* spp. than against *Anopheles* spp. There are conflicting reports regarding its efficacy against ticks.

DEET is undoubtedly useful in preventing the penetration of cercariae into the skin, but at best it should be regarded as an unreliable preventive against schistosomiasis.

2. A. DEET blocks odour receptors situated on the mosquito antennae. It thereby prevents a major way by which mosquitoes are attracted to humans. Knockdown repellents, e.g. many aerosol repellents, unlike DEET, kill insects as they fly. Although the effectiveness of DEET in terms of duration of action increases log-wise as the strength increases, to use more than 30–50% is counterproductive as allergic reactions and skin damage increase greatly at higher concentrations. DEET may reduce the potency of chemical sun blockers but the reverse does not hold true.

A study from Canada's University of Manitoba warns against using DEET-based mosquito repellents with sunblock. When a 2.5% solution of DEET was mixed with oxybenzone, a very common sunblocking ingredient, the amount of DEET absorbed into the skin went from 9.6% to 30.2%. There is some evidence that if sunblock and DEET are used together there may be an increased risk for stroke, headache, and hypertension.

3. D. Permethrin is a synthetic pyrethroid knockdown insecticide derived from a chemical found in the chrysanthemum family of plants. It is only used on clothes/nets and is made ineffective by the oils on our skin. It is effective for about 12 weeks. Permethrin is far superior to DEET against ticks.

4. B. Icaridin (Bayrepel®, Autan®) is a safe non-toxic repellent effective against a wide range of ticks, flies, midges, and mosquitoes, including *An. gambiae*, an important vector of malaria in Africa. It is as effective as DEET against mosquitoes and will not damage clothes or plastic.

5. A. Lemon eucalyptus (active component p-menthane-3,8-diol) is a natural repellent with proven efficiency and a nice smell. It is not as good as DEET or Icaridin. Other natural repellents include aniseed oil, cinnamon oil, thyme oil, nutmeg, and lavender oil.

It is convenient to separate those who differ from the general travelling population into easily identifiable categories or special groups. Each of these groups will require advice, medication, or vaccines that are tailored for their specific needs. Thus, the pregnant traveller must be warned of the increased risk of air-travel-related venous thrombosis, the diabetic of the danger of poor glycaemic control, and the young (male) traveller of the risks of casual sex. While there are very few people for whom overseas travel is absolutely contraindicated, common sense should always be heeded.

Pregnancy

1. **Which of the following is true regarding air travel and pregnancy?**
   A. There is an increased risk of premature labour
   B. Six transatlantic flights in 1 month significantly exceeds the acceptable level of radiation exposure
   C. Low molecular weight heparin is strongly contraindicated
   D. Venous thromboembolism (VTE) is a major potential hazard

2. **Which of the following is contraindicated in pregnancy?**
   A. Pneumococcal vaccine
   B. MMR (measles/mumps/rubella)
   C. Hepatitis A
   D. Influenza vaccine

3. **Which of the following is inexcusable to give to a pregnant woman?**
   A. Inactivated viral vaccine
   B. Inactivated bacterial vaccine
   C. Tetanus toxoid
   D. OPV

4. **PPD/tuberculin skin testing (Mantoux test)**
   A. Is interpreted the same, irrespective of whether pregnant or not
   B. May have an adverse effect on the foetus in the first trimester
   C. Is more likely to give a false-positive reaction in pregnancy
   D. May produce adverse effects in the mother

5. **Which of these is most likely to be teratogenic?**
   A. Mefloquine
   B. Proguanil
   C. Tetracyclines
   D. Pyrimethamine-sulfadoxine ('Fansidar' 25/500)

6. **Appropriate chemoprophylaxis for a woman who is 2 months pregnant and going to East Africa is**
   A. Chloroquin and proguanil
   B. Chloroquin alone
   C. Mefloquine
   D. No chemoprophylaxis

7. **The choice for ESBE of malaria in pregnancy is**
   A. Mefloquine
   B. ACT (artemisinin combined treatment, e.g. dihydroartemisinin/piperaquine, artemether/lumefantrine)
   C. Doxycycline
   D. Atovaquone/proguanil (Malarone™)

8. **For the chemoprophylaxis of malaria in pregnancy, in a chloroquin-sensitive area, use**
   A. Chloroquin at half the adult dose, in the first trimester
   B. Chloroquin at the full adult dose, irrespective of stage of pregnancy
   C. Mefloquine at full dose, irrespective of the trimester
   D. Atovaquone/proguanil in the second and third trimesters

9. **The CDC favours which of these during the first trimester in a highly malarious area?**
   A. Atovaquone/Proguanil (Malarone™)
   B. Mefloquine
   C. Doxycycline
   D. Only personal protective measures

10. **Quinine-induced hypoglycaemia occurs more frequently and is more serious when treating malaria in**
    A. Patients with HIV
    B. The elderly
    C. Pregnancy
    D. Diabetics

11. **Anopheline mosquitoes are more attracted to**
    A. Pregnant than to non-pregnant women
    B. Children than to adults
    C. Those with HIV than to others
    D. Men rather than to women (assume equal size and activity)

12. Suggested waiting times before becoming pregnant after
  A. Mefloquine is 3 months
  B. Atovaquone/proguanil is 2 months
  C. Doxycycline is 1 month
  D. Chloroquine is 6 months

13. Which of these would you be quite happy to give to a pregnant traveller?
  A. Bismuth subsalicicylate
  B. Probiotics
  C. DEET (50%)
  D. Co-trimoxazole (trimethoprim and sulfamethoxazole)

14. Which of the following is true for motion sickness in pregnancy?
  A. It is very rare
  B. Antihistamines are absolutely contraindicated
  C. Pyridoxine (vitamin B6) is absolutely contraindicated
  D. Ginger powder mixed with tea may help

15. Safe activities in pregnancy include
  A. Cross-country skiing
  B. Water skiing
  C. Sauna bathing
  D. Regular hot-tub baths

16. Acceptable activities in pregnancy include
  A. Air travel after the 38th week
  B. Commercial sea cruise at any time
  C. Mountain climbing up to 4580 m (15,000 feet)
  D. Use of permethrin on clothing

17. Which type of hepatitis has the highest mortality in pregnancy?
  A. Hepatitis A
  B. Hepatitis B
  C. Hepatitis C
  D. Hepatitis E

18. Which do you consider is the most serious cause of traveller's diarrhoea (TD) in a pregnant woman?
  A. Enterotoxigenic E. coli (ETEC)
  B. Listeria monocytogenes
  C. Norovirus
  D. Excess fruit/vegetables

Children

1. **Infants are less sensitive than adults to**
   A. Changes in altitude
   B. Changes in fluid status
   C. Ultraviolet irradiation
   D. Motion sickness

2. **An 8-month-old formula-fed infant is usually protected by maternal antibodies from**
   A. Rubella
   B. Measles
   C. Polio
   D. Tetanus

3. **Measles vaccine should be given to a travelling infant at**
   A. <3 months
   B. 3–6 months
   C. 6–12 months
   D. 12–15 months

4. **Which is most suitable for a 2–6-month-old child?**
   A. Meningococcal vaccine (polysaccharide)
   B. Typhoid (parenteral) vaccine
   C. Pneumococcal polysaccharide vaccine (23-valent)
   D. Pneumococcal conjugate vaccine (7-valent).

5. **Which of these is a contraindication to swimming in a child?**
   A. A recent history of an asthmatic attack
   B. A recently diagnosed mitral valve prolapse (MVP)
   C. A current 'swimmer's ear'
   D. Grommets in one or both ears

6. **Which of these is more likely in a child than in an adult?**
   A. Rabies
   B. Hepatitis A
   C. Japanese encephalitis
   D. Typhoid

7. **Which of the following diseases is usually very mild in a 2-year-old child?**
   A. Hepatitis A
   B. Meningitis
   C. Rabies
   D. Typhoid

8. **Which of the following is far more serious in a child than in an adult?**
   A. Dengue
   B. Malaria
   C. Japanese encephalitis
   D. Brucellosis

9. **Which of the following is true for TD in children?**
   A. It is rare in those less than 3 years old
   B. Oral rehydration is ineffective if the child is vomiting profusely
   C. Azithromycin is an antibiotic of choice for children with TD
   D. Acetazolamide has been found useful in correcting pH changes in acute TD in children

10. **If parenteral fluids must be given to a very severely dehydrated child the route of choice for the non-expert is**
    A. Intravenous
    B. Intraperitoneal
    C. Subcutaneous
    D. Intraosseous

11. **The dose of antivenom administered to a small child after a snake bite**
    A. Should be based on the age of the child
    B. Should be based on the length of time since being bitten
    C. Should be given in adult dosage
    D. Varies depending on what part of the body was bitten

The elderly

1. **Healthy elderly travellers are more likely than young adults to suffer from**
   A. TD
   B. Motion sickness
   C. Altitude sickness
   D. Hyperthermia

2. **Which of the following is true regarding yellow fever and the elderly?**
   A. Adverse reactions to yellow fever vaccination occur at about the same frequency as in young adults
   B. Yellow fever is a milder disease in the elderly
   C. Death from yellow fever is more likely in a non-immune elderly person than in a non-immune young person
   D. It is ethical to give a medical waiver whether there is informed consent or not to a 75-year-old who will spend <48 hours in a yellow fever destination, provided the likelihood of vaccine-associated adverse effects outweighs the threat of getting the disease

3. **Which of the following is true when comparing elderly to younger travellers?**
   A. The elderly have much the same sensitivity to sunlight
   B. The elderly have fewer problems with jet lag
   C. The elderly have much the same susceptibility to cold
   D. The elderly have a greater propensity for electrolyte and fluid imbalance

4. **The most common cause for an outbreak of diarrhoea on a cruise ship is**
   A. ETEC
   B. Salmonella
   C. Shigella
   D. Norovirus

Diabetics

1. **Diabetics should**
   A. Bring an adequate supply of their own insulin for stays longer than 1 month in a tropical country
   B. Ensure that their insulin is kept in a fridge at all times
   C. Check in advance that they can get the correct insulin in the host country
   D. Reduce their intake of fluids to a minimum during flights

2. **Insulin-dependent diabetics should**
   A. Transport insulin and syringes in cargo luggage for fear of problems with hand luggage examination and customs hassle at a foreign port of entry
   B. Reduce their usual insulin dosage by one-third if crossing three time zones or more
   C. Take their usual insulin dosage and schedule irrespective of the length of the journey
   D. Check blood sugar levels every 6 hours

3. **Most glucometers**
   A. Are accurate at altitudes below 20,880 m (60,000 feet)
   B. Read higher when above 3048 m (10,000 feet) than in a reference laboratory at ground level
   C. Read erroneously lower for every 304.8 m (1000 feet) one ascends from sea level
   D. Are little influenced by temperature or relative humidity

Asplenics

1. **The frequency of splenic damage after abdominal trauma in a western country is approximately**
   A. 1 in 4
   B. 1 in 40
   C. 1 in 400
   D. 1 in 4000

2. **Death from overwhelming infection in asplenic individuals compared to the general population is probably increased**
   A. 2-fold
   B. 10-fold
   C. 100-fold
   D. 6000-fold

3. **Death from sepsis in asplenic patients is most likely due to**
   A. Streptococcal infections
   B. Pneumococcal infections
   C. Multiple resistant *Staphylococcus aureus* (MRSA)
   D. Fulminant anaerobic infection

4. **The most common cause of overwhelming post-splenectomy sepsis (OPSS) is**
   A. *Streptococcus pneumoniae*
   B. *Streptococcus pyogenes*
   C. *Neisseria meinigitidis*
   D. Gram-negative septicaemia

5. **OPPS**
   A. Is most common in children
   B. Is most common 5–10 years post splenectomy
   C. Is unusual after splenectomy for spontaneous splenic rupure
   D. Carries a mortality approaching 10%

6. **The asplenic traveller**
   A. Is at greatly increased risk of contracting malaria
   B. Should avoid live vaccines
   C. Responds very poorly to polysaccharide vaccines
   D. Has enough splenic tissue remaining to provide useful function after a splenectomy for trauma

7. **Asplenic patients**
    A. Should only be given polysaccharide vaccines
    B. Are at greater risk than normal of contracting severe babesiosis
    C. Need vaccination against pneumococci at least 2 months before any major operation
    D. Commonly experience side effects after any combined vaccine

8. **A live viral vaccine may be given in**
    A. Asplenia
    B. HIV infection (symptomatic)
    C. Pregnancy
    D. Active immunosuppression following a bone transplant

Last-minute travellers

1. **Which of the following is true for last-minute travellers who make only one visit to the travel clinic?**
    A. Only give mandatory vaccines as required by International Health Regulations
    B. Give first doses of all required vaccines
    C. Recommend vaccination overseas by reputable person
    D. Carry vaccines overseas (keeping refrigerated)

2. **Which of the following is true regarding yellow fever vaccine and the last-minute traveller?**
    A. A certificate will be accepted up to the date of entry provided it is for a second or subsequent vaccination
    B. The certificate should be backdated so that entry to a yellow fever country is possible
    C. Only backdate the certificate if the traveller promises to stay in a city for at least the first 10 days
    D. Give a medical waiver if the traveller is only going away for a few days

Corporate and frequent travellers

1. **General advice to corporate travellers**
    A. Give SBET if going to a malarious area
    B. Advise they bring an antibiotic in case they get TD
    C. Advise they have locks on all luggage
    D. Advise they separate money into different pockets

2. **Frequent flyers and seafarers should be**
   A. Provided with a supply of antibiotics
   B. Given SBET for malaria if visiting endemic areas frequently
   C. Given repeated doses of live vaccines at 5-year intervals
   D. Informed specifically about the danger of sexually transmitted infections (STIs)

3. **Which of these factors contributes most to psychological stress in frequent international travellers?**
   A. Sleep deprivation
   B. Sense of isolation while overseas
   C. Over-indulgence in alcohol
   D. Workload faced on return home

Urban versus rural holidays

1. **Which of these statements conforms to the usual disease pattern?**
   A. Yellow fever is more likely in urban areas
   B. Diseases transmitted by *Ae. aegypti* are more frequent in rural areas
   C. Malaria is most unlikely if staying in a city hotel in tropical developing countries
   D. Cutaneous leishmaniasis is mainly a rural hazard

2. **Which of these is typically an 'urban' disease?**
   A. Japanese encephalitis vitus
   B. Bartonella (Carrions disease, Oroya fever)
   C. Chagas disease
   D. Dengue fever

3. **The most important hazard in large crowded cities is**
   A. Meningococcal meningitis
   B. Motor vehicle accidents
   C. Robbery
   D. Severe psychological stress

4. **A rural environment is more likely to be associated with**
   A. Contaminated water
   B. Ozone inhalation
   C. STIs
   D. Heat-related illness

Missionaries and expatriates

The term 'expatriate' refers to those who live abroad for many months or years. It includes long-term travellers, diplomats, technical experts, field researchers, health care personnel, humanitarian and development workers, and religious missionaries.

1. **Which of the following is most true of expatriates?**
   A. Expatriates are likely to have a similar number of health problems whether living in Africa or in India
   B. Expatriates are more likely than humanitarian workers to be involved in road traffic accidents
   C. Expatriates are more conscientious in taking malarial prophylaxis than routine travellers
   D. Expatriates are more likely to retire due to ill-health than their counterparts at home

Pilgrims and mass gatherings

There are special vaccination requirements needed to enter Saudi Arabia for the Hajj and Umra pilgrimages as well as for working in the Kingdom. These include proof of vaccination with OPV at least 6 weeks prior to entry if coming from a polio re-infected country, quadrivalent meningitis vaccination within 3 years and yellow fever vaccine from several non-endemic as well as all endemic countries. A list of regulations is available online or from any Saudi embassy.

1. **What is the most common medical problem at mass gatherings?**
   A. Influenza-like illness (ILI)
   B. Lack of medical facilities
   C. Diarrhoea
   D. Trauma

2. **Which of the following is important in prevention of ILI?**
   A. Wearing a face mask some of the time
   B. Wearing a face mask all the time
   C. Good personal hygiene
   D. Influenza vaccinations

3. **Which of the following is most true of illness outbreaks during the Hajj?**
   A. Up to one in ten pilgrims gets ill
   B. The risk of contracting hepatitis is negligible
   C. Heat stress is common even in wintertime
   D. Hospital admission is greatest in younger age groups

4. **Which of the following is most true of Hepatitis and the Hajj?**
   A. Hepatitis A is often acquired by pilgrims from drinking unsafe water
   B. Hepatitis B is virtually absent from the Hajj sites (Mecca, Medina, and Mina)
   C. Hepatitis C is virtually absent from Hajj sites
   D. Arboviral hepatitis has been eliminated

5. **Which of the following is most true of HIV and the Hajj?**
   A. Carrying anti-retroviral therapy (ART) across international borders may be difficult
   B. Compliance with ART is better during the pilgrimage than at other times
   C. Suboptimal adherence to ART for a week's pilgrimage has few if any deleterious consequences
   D. Hajj pilgrims have poorer adherence to ART than non-pilgrim visitors to Saudi-Arabia

Visiting friends and relatives

1. **Which of the following is a comprehensive definition of VFRs?**
   A. Recent immigrants who return to their ancestral country to visit friends, immediate family, or other relatives for a period of under 6 weeks
   B. Immigrants who return to their country of birth to stay with friends, immediate family, or other relatives irrespective of the length of stay
   C. Immigrants ethnically and racially distinct from the majority population of their country of current residence who return to their homeland
   D. Those, regardless of race or legal status, who travel abroad to visit friends or relatives and for whom there is a gradient of epidemiological risk between home and destination

2. **Failure of VFRs to visit a travel clinic before departure is mostly due to**
   A. The cost of attendance
   B. A generally poorer education than the majority of travellers
   C. Linguistic barriers
   D. Underestimation of risks

3. **Which is the most vulnerable group of VFRs?**
   A. Young adults (20–30 years of age)
   B. Children
   C. Women
   D. The elderly

Disabled travellers

1. **Which of the following is true regarding specific disabilities?**
   A. Visual impairment: guide dogs are admitted everywhere provided they are accompanied by a satisfactory vet's certificate
   B. Hearing loss: traveller must inform airline at least 48 hours in advance
   C. Mental impairment: mild cases may travel alone provided airline informed
   D. Mobility impaired: remove acid batteries from electric wheelchairs

2. **When travelling with guide dogs/service dogs**
   A. Feed the dog immediately before travel
   B. Sedate the dog before travel
   C. The dog's collar should include the date of latest rabies injection
   D. A metallic non-removable collar is essential

Pregnancy

1. D. Pregnancy-associated hypercoagulability and the impedance of venous return to the heart by a gravid uterus increase the chances of air-related VTE. Obesity is a compounding factor. There is no evidence that the risk of pre-term labour or miscarriage is increased. In any event about 7% of all pregnancies end in pre-term labour. Low-molecular-weight heparin is quite in order, especially if there is an extra risk of VTE, e.g. history of thrombophilia. Fifty milliremes per month is an acceptable level of radiation in pregnancy. One transatlantic flight exposes a person to about 4 milliremes.

2. B. MMR is a live vaccine. In exceptional circumstances live rubella vaccine can be given if the woman is non-immune and in a high-risk situation. Herpes vaccine (far greater dose of virus than varicella) is currently absolutely contraindicated at all stages of pregnancy. BCG vaccine is also contraindicated, although it is recorded that when live varicella vaccine was given inadvertently to 56 pregnant women there were no foetal or maternal adverse effects. Likewise no adverse effects have been found in foetus or mother after the inadvertent administration of live measles or mumps vaccines.

3. D. It is hard to envisage any circumstance in which OPV (live virus) should be given to a pregnant woman where damage to the foetus is a possibility. In addition to this immunological hyporesponsivness in pregnancy dampens the response to all vaccines. In practice most prefer to avoid any vaccinations in pregnancy unless deemed absolutely necessary.

4. A. The Mantoux test should be performed and interpreted exactly as in the non-pregnant woman.

5. C. Tetracyclines are the only currently used anti-malarials most likely to have teratogenic effects, although even this is in doubt (see question 9). Teratogenicity in humans has not been tested for the other options. However, in general one should avoid all drugs in the first trimester, unless absolutely necessary.

6. A. Although the efficacy of chloroquin and proguanil prophylaxis in East Africa is less than 50%, long usage has shown that they are well tolerated and do not cause foetal damage. Because proguanil inhibits dihydrofolate reductase, folate supplementation is more important than usual to prevent neural tube defects in the foetus. One can switch to mefloquine when the woman enters her second trimester.

Protection against non-falciparum types of malaria is also important and one cannot overstress personal protective measures should the woman make an informed judgment to visit East Africa.

7. B. ACT has replaced quinine as an SBET even in pregnancy. If possible, travel to high-risk malaria areas should be avoided in pregnancy because malaria tends to be more severe in pregnant women and maternal death, miscarriage, and foetal abnormalities are more common. Mefloquine can be used after the first trimester but no certainty exists regarding Malarone™. The drug used for SBET should be different from the one used in prophylaxis and no resistance should have been found against it in the country in question. The concept of SBET without regular chemopropylaxis is gaining support among many travel medicine physicians.

8. B. Give chloroquine in adult dosage (500 mg salt or 300 mg base) once a week. Start 1–2 weeks before departure and continue for 4 weeks after return. Avoid chloroquine where there are the usual contraindications (alcoholism, liver disease, psoriasis, hypersensitivity to 4-aminoquinolines).

Mefloquine is believed to be safe in the second and third trimesters. The effects of Malarone® (atovaquone/proguanil) in pregnancy are not known, although the benefits may outweigh the side effects if no other antimalarial is deemed effective and if the woman must travel to a highly malarious area where chloroquine resistance is found.

9. B. The CDC permits the use of mefloquine during all stages of pregnancy. Teratogenicity using high doses in animals is most unlikely to be applicable to humans.

Data on Malarone is scarce and although the proguanil component is considered safe, the protective effects of atovaquone may not outweigh any potential danger, however remote.

Studies from several sources now indicate that foetal malformations are not more common in pregnant women who take tetracyclines at any stage of pregnancy (Hellgren and Rombo 2010). Recall too that staining of the offspring's permanent teeth has never been reported after using doxycycline in pregnancy.

10. C. Quinine-induced hypoglycemia comes on very rapidly and more frequently in patients who are pregnant. The warning signs are fits, abnormal behaviour, and a change in the level of consciousness.

11. A. Pregnant women attract twice the number of *Anopheles gambiae*—the predominant vectors of malaria in Africa—than their non-pregnant counterparts. This is probably due to physiological changes associated with pregnancy that attract mosquitoes (increased heat, sweat, CO_2 production). Oestrogens, lactic acid, urea, perfumes, and dark colours are among other factors that attract mosquitoes. Any perceived preference to bite men is based on mens' larger size and greater CO_2 production. Having said all that, there is another way of looking at the attraction for mosquitoes in pregnancy: perhaps it is only those mosquitoes that actually carry *P. falciparum* that find pregnant women more attractive than anyone else.

12. A. The following are suggested waiting times: mefloquine 3 months, atovaquone/proguanil 2 weeks, doxycycline 1 week, chloroquin no contraindication (P Schlagenhauf, Boston 2011).

13. B. So far probiotics have proved harmless to both mother and foetus. Bismuth may possibly be associated with CNS symptoms in the baby; high-dose DEET with foetal toxicity (rare and ? due to misuse); co-trimoxazole with a single case of neutropenia in the baby.

14. D. Non-prescription remedies such as ginger powder and pyridoxine are often stated to be helpful.

Motion sickness is not rare and may be confused with morning sickness.

Antihistamines are also used and have no more side effects than in the non-pregnant state. Lomotil™ should not be used. Scopolamine can cause foetal arrhythmias.

15. A. Gentle cross-country skiing is acceptable but downhill skiing is not because of the possibility of a stressful tachycardia. Similarly, surface swimming is strongly recommended while water skiing, diving or scuba diving are not (infection via water entering vagina).

Hot tubs and saunas cause hyperthermia and can also be a source of infection.

16. D. Nets and clothing impregnated with permethrin and the use of repellents such as DEET (<25%) or picaridin (<10%) are safe in pregnancy.

Airlines discourage travel after about 35 weeks although travel in pressurized cabins (5000–8000 feet or 1500–2400 m) is without adverse effect on a healthy mother or her unborn. A doctor's letter is needed by some airlines for short-haul travel up to 32 weeks and long-haul up to 28 weeks.

Cruise ship companies usually refuse boarding to women >28 weeks pregnant because of the dangers of motion sickness, falls in bad weather, sea sickness, and limited on-board obstetric facilities.

Visiting locations >10,000 feet may induce acute mountain sickness, sickling in susceptible women, and hypothermia if there is much exposure to outside conditions.

17. D. Mortality in pregnancy for hepatitis E is usually greater than 20%. Hepatitis E has reached epidemic proportions in many developing countries in recent times. It is transmitted in the same way as hepatitis A.

18. B. Listeriosis is common and serious in pregnancy, especially in the last trimester, when the mother's immune system is at its lowest. Fatalities occur and stillbirth is frequent (22%).

Listeriosis, so-called after Lord Lister, is due to a motile Gram-positive bacillus common in food, especially in meat, milk, and cheese. Toxoplasmosis is also a major threat and is associated with foetal stillbirth and foetal abnormalities. *E. coli* and norovirus also occur but are generally not as serious.

Fruits and vegetables stimulate the bowels and if diarrhoea occurs the BRAT diet (banana, rice, apple sauce, toast) may help. If so, be sure to supplement with folate and minerals, e.g. zinc.

Children

1. D. Motion sickness is rare before the age of 2 years and increases to a maximum by the age of 12 years. Infants are more sensitive than adults to changes in altitude, fluid status, and UV irradiation. A healthy full-term infant may travel in modern aircraft although some recommend that they should not travel by air if <7 days old.

2. B. Antibodies to measles usually persist in the infant from birth to 15 months. Most other passively transferred antibodies are gone at 4–6 months. Since antibodies are mainly transferred in the last trimester of pregnancy the premature infant is more at risk of a variety of diseases.

3. C. A satisfactory response to measles vaccine can be expected at 6–12 months of age. Below 6 months the response is poor because of the high level of maternal antibody in the baby.

4. D. The serogroups of the 7-valent conjugate pneumococcal vaccine (Prevnar®), which are frequent causes of illness in young children, are often resistant to penicillin. A newer 13-valent conjugate vaccine is now used. This protects against the most invasive pneumococci. It is given to children aged 6 weeks to 5 years and to those <18 years who are clearly at-risk.

For children, a good schedule is to give the vaccine at 2, 4, and 12 months.

The 23-valent polysaccharide form is suitable for children over 2 years of age.

Meningococcal and typhoid vaccines are poorly immunogenic in those under 2 years old.

5. D. Any perforation of the tympanic membrane, whether by disease or by tympanoplasty, allows water to enter the middle ear when swimming. Other contraindications to swimming include a long QTc >500 ms, a confirmed history of epilepsy, and any previous episode of loss of consciousness when in water. Most MVPs are symptomless and pose no particular hazard for the child who is swimming. Swimmer's ear (otitis externa) is no obstacle. It should be treated with routine topical medications.

6. A. Children are fascinated by animals and in some areas up to 40% of rabies cases occur in under 14-year-olds. While hygiene standards are understandably low in a small child, nonetheless accompanying adults usually take great care to ensure children only ingest clean food and water when on holiday overseas. This helps avoid hepatitis A and typhoid. Similar concern ensures that children are protected from mosquito bites.

7. A. Hepatitis A is usually very mild in children. Any of the other three options can be deadly serious. Faeces are swarming with HAV in children who have active infection, therefore should a small child contract hepatitis A, the live virus will be easily spread to adult minders and other children, perhaps on return home.

8. B. Malaria occurs more quickly and may be rapidly life-threatening in children. Only pregnant women, those with asplenia, and seriously debilitated people get malaria as badly.

Chloroquin, mefloquine, and atovaquone/proguanil are all acceptable prophylactics for children when given in recommended dosage. Doxycycline can be given to those over at least 8 years of age. However, the rationale behind the current prohibition of doxycycline in chidren is disputed. So far no tooth discoloration has been documented in humans after doxycycline. Remember that tooth development takes place during the last half of pregnancy.

9. C. TD is common in children<3 years of age and ORS is the mainstay of treatment even if the child is vomiting. Patience and persistence must be exercised. Parenteral fluid will be needed in severe cases.

Azithromycin (10 mg/kg po qid × 3 days) or ciprofloxacin (10 mg/kg/day po) are both useful in children, but it is impossible to label any specific antibiotic as being the one of choice in all cases. Acetazolamide causes acidosis and should be avoided.

10. D. Intra-osseous administration of fluids is simple and efficient, and can rehydrate the child sufficiently so that other routes, preferably the oral route, can be used. Intra-peritoneal infusions are suitable for use in very large outbreaks of dehydration, e.g. in famines and refugee camps where clinics are inundated with cases. The IV route may seem ideal but finding a vein in a dehydrated, often moribund child can be very challenging and waste precious time. Subcutaneous fluids are of limited value, have uncertain absorption, and are painful.

11. C. Figure this out for yourself!

The elderly

1. D. Thermoregulation, in particular vasodilation and sweating, is impaired in the elderly and they cannot cope with heat like a younger person can. Antihypertensive drugs that impair sympathoreflexes and diuretics that lower the intravascular volume compound the problem.

Although factors favouring TD such as achlorhydria (>40% over 65 years), being on proton pump inhibitors, or suffering from irritable bowel syndrome, and are common in the elderly, young people are far more prone to take risks with food and thus TD is more frequent in the young.

Motion sickness becomes less of a problem for the elderly. There appears to be no relation per se between age and altitude sickness.

2. C. Yellow fever is a more serious and deadly disease in the elderly. At the same time adverse reactions to yellow fever vaccination increase sharply with age. Immunity, as measured by antibody levels, is less and slower to achieve in the elderly. A serious adverse event occurs 11.6 times more often in those over 75 years than in 25–44-year-olds. Despite the best of intentions one should never give a waiver without the informed and written consent of the patient. Remember that several countries, e.g. Egypt, South Africa, Tanzania, and India, can demand proof of yellow fever vaccination even after transit in technically yellow fever-free countries such as Kenya, Zambia, and Uganda.

3. D. The older person copes with fluid and electrolyte loss poorly compared to the younger person. The older person may well have increased sensitivity to sunlight due to being on drugs such as sulphas, oral hypoglycaemics, NSAIDS, diuretics, or tetracyclines. Susceptibility to jet lag and hypothermia is greater in the elderly.

4. D. Many elderly people take sea cruises. Norovirus (Norwalk virus, 'vomiting bug') is the most common cause of acute gastrointestinal illness in cruise ships and is also a very common cause in closed environments such as hospitals, nursing homes, homes for the elderly, restaurants, and schools.

Norovirus can be spread via food, fomites, and person-to-person. Control is difficult despite isolation, hand washing, and good personal hygiene. One study has shown that rigorous and repeated cleaning of public toilet areas is associated with a decrease in the number of outbreaks. People with blood group B (more common in Asians) are more resistant to Norovirus than others.

Diabetics

1. C. It is important to be sure of a continuous supply of the same or compatible insulin, and long-term travellers should organize this in advance. Insulin will keep out of a fridge for 1 month provided the temperature range is between 2 and 30°C. Most fridge temperatures range from 2 to 8°C but this range is by no means assured in many countries where frequent power outages occur.

It is important to keep fully hydrated while flying. Dehydration can lead to thermoregulation problems as well as render glucose monitoring more difficult.

2. D. The ability to check blood sugar regularly is essential for the travelling diabetic whose meal schedule and type is altered and who is under the stress that accompanies travel. Keep insulin in hand luggage for ease of access, in case cargo luggage goes astray, and because the temperature in the cargo bay may affect the potency of insulin. If crossing five time zones or less routine insulin schedules should be used.

3. C. Most glucometers underestimate blood glucose levels at altitudes of >2000 m (6500 feet). This fact is important for diabetics who ski or trek at high altitudes or fly in commercial jets. It is important to know how your glucometer performs and whether it is a GOX (glucose oxidase) or GDH (glucose dehydrogenase) based machine. As temperature and relative humidity rise many glucometers record false low values for blood glucose. The lack of accuracy and consistency in the performance of most glucometers >2000 m should be known by diabetic patients who live in or intend to ascend to high altitude.

Asplenics

1. A. One in four suffer splenic damage after abdominal trauma (Level 1 Trauma Centres USA, 2009). This rate is probably higher in parts of the world where pre-existing splenic pathology is prevalent, e.g with malaria, S. mansoni.

2. C.

3. B. Most cases succumb to pneumococcal infection, although other encapsulated bacteria also pose increased risks, e.g. H. influenza and N. meningitidis.

4. A. Overall, S. pneumonia is the major infectious cause of death in humans. In OPSS it accounts for over 90% of cases. The other organisms listed are of major importance in the remaining 10% of cases. Note that bites from healthy dogs and cats, whose saliva contains the sometimes deadly Gram-negative bacterium C. canimorsus, can also cause OPPS. Some tropical bacteria and protozoal organisms are reported to be more common in asplenic people, e.g. S. typhi, leishmania, trypanosoma.

5. A. OPPS carries a mortality of over 50% and is most common and most deadly in children. In all cases the greatest risk is in the first year after loss of splenic function but the threat is life-long.

Methods to prevent OPPS include the conservative treatment of splenic rupture and the use of prophylactic antibiotics plus routine vaccinations that include pneumococcal vaccine. Large spleens rupture readily.

6. C. Despite a poor response to polysaccharide vaccines every effort should be made to fully immunize the asplenic traveller, including the use of live vaccines.

Although disputed, there is no proved association between malaria and asplenia, and there is no reason why malaria should occur more frequently. However, if malaria occurs then it is more likely to be fatal in the asplenic person and animal models suggest that asplenia exacerbates malaria.

One can expect useful function to be retained after splenectomy for trauma only if there are large or numerous accessory spleens retained. Note that asplenia includes functional as well as anatomical asplenia.

7. B. There is a well-established association between asplenia and the severity of babesiosis. Babesiosis is an uncommon tick-borne protozoal zoonosis with fewer than 400 human cases reported. It is similar clinically to malaria and may be treated with quinine/clindaymcin or atovaquone/azithromycin. Mortality of up to 43% has been recorded. Note, however, that babesiosis already is the most frequently reported infection transmitted through transfusion in the USA and in New York City alone in 2009 six transfusion-associated cases of babesiosis were reported. There is no proved association between the severity of influenza and asplenia. OPSS is more likely in children and in those who had splenectomy in childhood. Routine vaccinations apply to all patients with asplenia, but the response to vaccination is likely to be reduced following splenectomy, particularly to polysaccharide vaccines. There is no special rule regarding vaccinations and major surgery.

8. A.

Last-minute travellers

1. B. All necessary vaccines can be given at separate sites on the same day without impairing antibody responses or increasing the rates of adverse reactions. If there is an opportunity for subsequent visits, shortened schedules (0, 7, 21 days) can be used for rabies, hepatitis A ,and hepatitis B immunizations. Unfortunately, in the case of vaccines needing more than one dose, the length of seroprotection provided by shortened schedules may be less than desired (CDC Yellow Book, 2012).

2. A. Legally a 10-day rule applies to the first yellow fever vaccination before it is accepted by the port health authority as valid for entry. However, a second or subsequent dose can be given within 24 hours of entry. Never backdate a certificate: this is medically, morally, and legally wrong.

Corporate and frequent travellers

1. D. Corporate travellers should be remined to keep money of different denominations in different pockets and make sure that small denomination billls are easy to access, e.g. for tipping, taxis, and incidentals. Passports, airline tickets, and other valuables should always be securely carried on one's person. Skillful robberies can be completed without the victim noticing. Locked luggage gives a false sense of security and can easily be opened without the owner noticing and without forcing the lock. It is also advisable never walk alone in a strange place, especially after dark.

Taxicabs, whether at the airport or on the street, can overcharge and even facilitate personal crime. Bus stations and markets are notorious locations for robberies and business people often fall victim to crime when making rushed last-minute buys. Loperamide is useful in mild cases of diarrhoea but should not be used as a prophylactic agent. Even proponents of standby treatment for malaria do not advise it for West Africa. Antibiotics should not be provided as a rule.

2. D. It is always wise to spend extra time explaining how easy it is to contract an STI. This applies to all travellers but especially to sex tourists, young adults, frequent flyers, and seafarers. Personal protective measures together with basic education about malaria is far more important than an unrealistic expectation or undue reliance on chemoprophylaxis. Expert help will usually be available either at the destination or at the home base.

Most live vaccines protect for life and a booster, if given, is normally done at 10-year intervals.

It is unwise to provide antibiotics to these travellers. The danger of incomplete courses, using them when not indicated or for trivial conditions, undue reliance on them when a visit to a doctor is more appropriate, and using them beyond their expiry date are the main reasons for this conservative approach.

3. D. Contemporary studies support the view that returning home to a very heavy workload is the greatest single stressor in frequent travellers.

One study, on 498 global business travellers for the World Bank, showed that a third of them reported high levels of travel stress. It seems logical to assume that the strain is even greater for those who travel in a less organized manner, e.g. those seeking business abroad or visiting politically or culturally hostile countries.

Urban versus rural holidays

1. D. Cutaneous leishmaniasis is still regarded as a rural disease, although foci of zoonotic cutaneous leishmaniasis have been reported from several cities in Colombia.

Ae. aegypti is a peridomestic mosquito and is common in cities. Should the balance tip, its presence may cause an explosion of yellow fever in hitherto untouched cities in South America. Urban malaria is well known and on the increase due to sprawling shanty towns with an abundance of mosquito breeding sites. In addition there is a huge commuter population in many cities, e.g. Mumbai and Chennai, that allows infected people to carry the parasite into their city work places every day.

2. D. Dengue fever is more likely in an urban than in a rural setting. Japanese encephalitis is primarily a rural disease. It is widespread in South-East Asia and India. However, nothing is straightforward! For example, dengue fever is rife in parts of rural Brazil and Argentina, and Japanese encephalitis vitus is not a problem in rural Brazil, although six flaviviruses, genetically related to Japanese encephalitis vitus, have been found there. Chagas disease (American trypanosomiasis) is transmitted by triatomine bugs and is primarily a rural disease. Bartonella bacilliformis is found in Peru, Ecuador, and Colombia, and, while rare, carries a mortality of over

90% in the acute phase. It is transmitted by sand flies. Other forms of bartonellosis are also rare, but less serious, e.g. cat scratch disease (*B. henselae*).

3. B. Motor vehicle accidents are the most common cause of death in travellers, especially in younger travellers. In Lagos, Nigeria, buses are known as 'flying coffins' and anyone who has tried to cross a busy road in places as diverse as Cairo, Bangalore, and Damascus will appreciate that the threat to life is very real. Contributory factors include poor driving, speed, badly maintained and overcrowded vehicles, lack of safe crossings, driving on different sides of the road, and fatigue-induced misjudgement by the traveller. The other options listed are also important considerations, particularly in cities.

4. A. There is little or no purification of water supplied by local authorities in rural areas but quite often drinking water is chlorinated and filtered in urban supplies.

Ground ozone levels are higher in cities because of the effect of sunlight on nitrogenous volatile organic compounds.

Ozone is an inflammatory agent that has been shown to increase respiratory disease, including asthma, in urban dwellers in proportion to its level in the atmosphere. Levels of carbon monoxide haemoglobin can go above 5% in city dwellers. This is a value that seriously compromises oxygen carriage in the blood. Other major pollutants in cities include NO_2, particulate matter, and lead.

STIs are rampant in commercial as well as non-commercial sex workers, and it is apparent that counselling before departure fails to restrain the sexual behaviour of most travellers. The typical sex tourist is male with a mean age of 38.

Temperatures in cities may be as much as 6°C higher than those found in the countryside. This is due to the 'hot dome' effect that occurs over large cities, where heat is absorbed and radiated from concrete and asphalt. This applies as much to cities such as London, New York, and Tokyo as to any megapolis in the developing world. However, the elderly tourist is a special risk (see above, sub-section Elderly travellers). Thirst is not always a reliable guide to body hydration.

Missionaries and expatriates

1. D. Studies on missionaries and long-term expatriates show that ill-health is a fairly common cause of early retirement. This is a mere generalization since the individual's response to the added stress, quality of living conditions, length of time overseas, local hazards and nature of the work all affect the outcome.

A study on Scottish Presbyterian Missionaries from 1867 to 1929 indicated that Africa was a more hazardous location to work in than India. This is still likely to be the case in regard to sub-Saharan Africa.

Road traffic accidents are more common in humanitarian workers, presumably because of their younger age.

Compliance with malarial chemoprophylaxis and the use of nets and sprays usually decreases over weeks and months, yet many long-term expatriates are extremely fastidious in this regard.

Pilgrims and mass gatherings

1. A. ILI is the most common. The CDC defines an ILI as cough and/or sore throat together with fever (>37.8°C) in the absence of a known cause other than influenza. A study by Gautret et al. on French pilgrims to the Hajj in 2007 showed that cough was by far the most common symptom (51%) followed by headaches (21.2%), heat stress (12.3%), fever (9.1%), diarrhoea (4.5%), vomiting (2.4%), injury (2.2%), and skin disease (1.1%).

There are first-class medical facilities available for Hajj pilgrims.

2. C. It is suggested that personal hygiene, e.g. covering the mouth when coughing, together with disinfectant hand rubs (non-alcoholic in the Hajj), is the most realistic way of reducing the number of ILIs.

It may be that facemasks are ineffective and that wearing them on and off is associated with the greater likelihood of upper respiratory infection and sore throat. Thin paper masks, wet masks, and re-used and shared masks may account for this.

The majority of reports show that influenza vaccination has little or no protective effect. This may be due to immunization by an influenza strain different to that prevailing at the gathering/pilgrimage.

While the Hajj is the largest pilgrimage on earth (more than 2.5 million pilgrims visit Mecca annually) there are many other places of mass gatherings, e.g. sporting events (the World Cup, Olympic Games) and pilgrimages (Buddhist, Christian, Jewish), which share these risks.

3. C. Heat-related stress occurs in >10% of pilgrims even during the winter months. This is due to the huge mass of pilgrims crowding into a relatively small space. Heat exhaustion and heat stroke are major problems during the summer months. The Saudi authorities have combated this by providing shaded roads, rest areas, clean drinking water, mist sprays, segregation of vehicles from pedestrians, and air-conditioned accommodation. Professor Nasr El Din did pioneering work in this regard in conjunction with the London School of Hygiene and Tropical Medicine.

4. A. Hepatitis A is the most common. It is transmitted via the faeco-oral route and via ingestion of viral contaminated food and water. To combat this, clean water is provided for all pilgrims and this has reduced the incidence dramatically.

Hepatitis B is a real risk from cuts received during head shaving at the end of the pilgrimage. Many unlicensed barbers ply their trade along the roadside and one study showed that 4% were HBsAg positive, of whom 20% were unaware of their condition. Sharing of razors and other utensils in crowded tents may also contribute to the spread of HBV. Recall that Saudi Arabia is a HBV-endemic country.

Hepatitis C antibody is found in 4.3% of blood donors in Saudi Arabia and is transmitted in a similar way to HBV.

Gargling and sharing of a toothbrush or dental floss with an HCV-infected person may cause transmission of the disease. Saliva contains HCV and one study elegantly demonstrated that HCV levels increase in saliva after teeth brushing. Devout Muslims brush their teeth before every prayer.

Alkhumra virus is a flavirus that was discovered in 1995. It is carried by a night-biting tick and may also be transmitted via camel milk. It causes a flu-like illness and hepatitis (100%), bleeding (55%), and encephalitis (20%). Although not common, it does occur and has a case fatality rate >30%. There is hope that a vaccine can be developed against this virus in the next 10 years.

5. A. Several countries routinely confiscate such medicines and may even deport the traveller. Saudi Arabia is particularly vigilant in this regard. Cultural, social, and religious reasons make adherence to ART difficult during the pilgrimage. Thus it is not surprising that compliance with ART is better in the pre- and post-travel periods than during the pilgrimage itself. In one study from Kano it was found that over two-thirds of HIV+ pilgrims missed their medications for patient-related reasons. Sub-optimal compliance with ART is serious both for the patient and for the emergence of resistant strains of the virus.

Visiting friends and relatives

1. D. This is a broad definition that many would accept. The epidemiological risks include socioeconomic status, genetic attributes, cultural risks, environmental exposures, and personal behaviour. This definition of VFRs is being further broadened nowadays to include subsequent generations who maintain a cultural identity with their country of origin.

VFRs constitute a high-risk group which needs special attention.

2. D. VFRs have low rates of attendance at pre-travel consultations. VFRs often consider that they have immunity to most diseases, e.g. malaria, typhoid, and hepatitis A, in their homeland. This belief is strengthened by talking to other VFRs who have returned to their host country and have encountered no health problems whatsoever while away. This belief is not true. Of the examples just given, only a previous attack of hepatitis A confers life-long immunity.

In a study from Quebec only 6% cited cost as a deterrent and in a US study 90% of VFRs to Asia had a college education.

3. B. Those under 20 years of age are almost certainly the most vulnerable. Reasons given are a failure to take precautions against common diseases, the practice of showing off children to extended family, allowing children to mix, play, and socialize unsupervised, and allowing them to caress animal pets. Children born to immigrants in their country of adoption should be protected in exactly the same way as native children when they travel abroad.

Disabled travellers

1. D. Wet batteries are not allowed and only dry batteries should be used. Travellers are advised to bring the lightest possible wheelchairs. All removable items must be taken off before the chair is stored. There is no extra cost for taking a wheelchair, stick, crutch or walking aid.

There are no legal hindrances to travel for mentally impaired people but common sense should prevail and an accompanying person may well be necessary. It is important that they carry ID showing their home and overseas contact numbers.

Many countries, especially island countries such as Australia, the UK, New Zealand, and Ireland, insist on long quarantine periods for guide dogs. This means that the traveller will be without this valuable help, perhaps for the duration of the proposed trip. Travellers should also understand the regulations covering the re-importation of their guide dogs to their home countries.

Deaf travellers are not subject to any special legal constraints, but they can ask airlines in advance to provide them with person-to-person information on pertinent announcements.

2. C. It is important to use a non-metallic collar, incorporating facts such as the last rabies shot, in case the dog scratches or bites someone. One should neither feed nor sedate the dog before travel, and every effort should be made to have the dog void before embarkation. The traveller should not ask for an aisle or emergency seat, for fear of obstructing the aisle.

Remember that guide dogs are service dogs and are not pets. This designation confers freedom of access to the dog wherever his or her master goes.

There has been a remarkable increase in adventure and extreme travel in recent years. This includes travel in remote areas, mountain climbing, e.g. Kilamanjaro, living in rough and dangerous situations, and working in slums and shanty towns. Young adults, students, and backpackers constitute the majority of adventure travellers. They also constitute a group that is the most careless about health and most loathe spending money on a pre-travel consultation.

Chapter 10 is devoted to special activities, which is a natural continuation of adventure travel.

General

1. **Which of the following do you consider the most important advice for a travel clinic to give?**
   A. Advise the traveller from personal experience
   B. Make sure that the traveller has adequate insurance
   C. Suggest a good internet site for the activity/destination proposed
   D. Provide the traveller with a standard travel medical kit

2. **The major problem for adventurers is**
   A. Relationship with companion(s)
   B. Not knowing the local language
   C. Loneliness
   D. Fear of the unknown

3. **Adventurers exposed to bat-infested caves are more likely than other tourists to be exposed to**
   A. Leptospirosis
   B. Endemic mycoses
   C. Anaerobic infections
   D. Bites from snakes

4. **Risk is most minimal with which of the following?**
   A. Henna tattoos in the Sudan
   B. Body piercing in a reputable holiday resort
   C. Herbal tea in Malawi
   D. Pharmacist advice in Thailand

Potable water

1. **The most reliable way to purify water is to**
   A. Boil it
   B. Use iodine tablets and let stand for 1 hour
   C. Chlorinate it to international standards
   D. Use filtration and iodination

2. **The cysts of Cryptosporidium are destroyed by**
   A. Iodine
   B. Chlorine
   C. Filtration
   D. Permethrin

3. **Water is made potable at sea level if boiled for at least**
   A. 1 minute
   B. 5 minutes
   C. 10 minutes
   D. 15 minutes

4. **The surest way to sterilize water is to**
   A. Expose it to ultraviolet irradiation
   B. Heat it
   C. Halogenate it (ensuring 3–5 mg residual halogen)
   D. Carry out a two-step filtration or coagulation/flocculation followed by halogenation

5. **To make water potable at 3048 m (10,000 feet) one should boil it for**
   A. 1 minute
   B. 3 minutes
   C. 10 minutes
   D. 20 minutes

6. **The addition of 50 mg of vitamin C (ascorbic acid) to 1 l of iodinated water**
   A. Makes the water taste better
   B. Is only effective if added before iodine is added
   C. Enhances the action of iodine
   D. Kills organisms against which iodine is ineffective

7. **Iodine (tablets or liquid)**
   A. Is a better water disinfectant than chlorine
   B. Can disinfect cloudy water (containing particulate matter)
   C. Needs contact with clear water at room temperature for about 10 minutes to be effective
   D. Needs contact with turbid water for 20 minutes at room temperature to be effective

8. **Halogenation of water with iodine or chlorine is**
   A. Effective against most viruses
   B. Effective against Cryptosporidium
   C. Effective against giardia
   D. Relatively expensive

9. **The three-dish strategy means that you**
   A. Have at least three people on any expedition to a remote area
   B. Make sure there are at least three meals each day
   C. Make sure there is a balance between protein, carbohydrate, and fat
   D. Wash dishes sequentially in three different bowls

10. **To make potable water with minimum equipment one should**
    A. Drink directly from natural springs
    B. Filter via clean cloth and allow to settle for 5 minutes
    C. Filter via any cloth and allow to settle for 10 minutes
    D. Add household bleach

Rafting

1. **Death among those kayaking or rafting in remote white waters is most commonly due to**
   A. Drowning
   B. Trauma
   C. Camp fire burns
   D. Dehydration/diarrhoea/exposure

2. **Swallowing or immersion in water while rafting in remote areas of Asia most commonly results in**
   A. Leptospirosis
   B. Schistosomiasis
   C. Heptatis A
   D. Giardiasis

3. **Leptospirosis**
    A. Is becoming less frequent in most countries
    B. Has now been reported from polar regions
    C. Is due to a highly motile spirochete
    D. Is easily diagnosed on a blood film

4. **The highest incidence of reported leptospirosis occurs in**
    A. Cuba
    B. Queensland
    C. The Seychelles
    D. Italy

Climate extremes

1. **Which of these is the most frequent in a polar expedition?**
    A. Injury
    B. Respiratory tract infection
    C. Musculo-skeletal problems
    D. Psychiatric disturbance

2. **Which of these is the most frequent in a polar expedition?**
    A. Sunburn
    B. Snow blindness
    C. Dental pain
    D. Frostbite

3. **Which environmentally related problem is most common in those travelling in cold areas?**
    A. Hypothermia
    B. Frostbite
    C. Snow blindness
    D. Trench foot

4. **Frostbite is most likely to occur if conditions are**
    A. Calm and dry
    B. Windy and dry
    C. Windy and wet
    D. Between 0 and 30°C

5. **Heat exhaustion is best prevented by**
   A. Wearing light-coloured clothes
   B. Wearing shorts
   C. Drinking copiously
   D. Using cooling devices such as fans

6. **In a hot environment**
   A. A nearly colourless urine indicates possible renal failure
   B. Alcohol slows acclimatisation
   C. Increasing the humidity facilitates acclimatisation
   D. Dosage of antihypertensives, e.g. β- or calcium-blockers, must be increased

7. **The most common cause of serious illness when exercising in a hot environment is**
   A. Lack of glucose
   B. Acidosis
   C. Hyperkalaemia
   D. Hyponatraemia

8. **The first priority In the treatment of heat exhaustion/heat stroke is**
   A. Placement of an IV line
   B. Oral salt replacement
   C. Putting ice packs around the torso
   D. Exposing the total body to alternate warm and cool water

Snakes and scorpions

1. **First aid after a snakebite to the leg should include**
   A. Immobilization of the entire affected limb
   B. Compression bandaging proximal to the bite to prevent spread of toxin
   C. A small incision and thorough washing out of the bite area
   D. Suction of the bite area

2. **Which of the following is true for envenomation?**
   A. A scorpion sting is never fatal
   B. Scorpion and spider stings together make up the bulk of venomous arthropod stings
   C. Elapids (cobras, kraits) account for the greatest number of deaths from snakebite in the tropics
   D. Vipers typically cause devastating local myonecrosis and CNS symptoms

3. **What percentage of people will develop signs of envenomation after being bitten by a poisonous snake?**
   A. <5%
   B. 25–50%
   C. 50–70%
   D. 70–100%

4. **Which of the following is true for snake envenomations?**
   A. Most deaths from snake bites occur in Africa
   B. Vipers account for most bites
   C. Children are more resistant to snake bites than adults
   D. Coral snakes are harmless

5. **Scorpion and spider stings are**
   A. Often unnoticed
   B. Less common than snake bites
   C. Associated with autonomic activation
   D. Less painful than snakebites

Marine envenomations and injuries

1. **Which of the following is true for box jellyfish stings in tropical waters?**
   A. The victim typically experiences multiple 'pin pricks'
   B. Death can occur in 2–3 minutes after a sting
   C. Sodium bicarbonate applied locally eases any pain
   D. The first reported fatality occurred in the 1990s

2. **After an attack by 'shockers' (electric rays and electric eels)**
   A. Usually no treatment is required
   B. Hot immersion is the treatment of choice
   C. There are fragments of the fish spine left in the victims skin
   D. Skin scales are often left in the victim's skin

War zones

1. **When travelling in a war zone it is most important to have**
   A. Several copies of one's passport
   B. Up to 12 passport-sized photos of yourself
   C. The address of the nearest friendly embassy
   D. Official ID from a neutral agency, e.g. ICRC, UNHCR

ADVENTURE TRAVELLERS

ANSWERS

General

1. B. All are important but arguably good insurance cover is the most important. Things may have changed since you made your trip, internet sites often plug their own agendas, and a standard medical kit may lull the traveller into a false sense of security. A fifth option, namely the ability to communicate with the outside world, is probably more important than any of those listed above.

2. A. Adventurers are intrepid characters with little fear of the unknown, the ability to manage in difficult situations, and self-belief in being able to surmount obstacles. However, all through history, the inability of explorers and adventurers to get along with companions is very striking and even today this is the greatest single problem among humanitarian volunteers.

3. B. Mycoses, particularly histoplasmosis and coccidioidomycosis, which exist throughout the world, are likely to be contracted even in young immunocompetent people who visit bat-infested caves or who do community service in endemic areas. Generally these mycoses present as acute febrile pulmonary infections but they may disseminate widely in immunocompromised people. Note that infection can occur when humans are exposed to dust, e.g. from a nearby construction site, even if they are staying in luxury hotels. Note also the possibility of bat rabies in caves.

4. D. Pharmacists are highly trained and reliable in Thailand.

Henna tatoos and any sort of body piercing should be avoided for fear of hepatitis B, HIV, or bacterial contamination. Hebal teas may contain toxic and hallucinogenic organic compounds.

Potable water

1. A. Adequate boiling is without doubt the most consistently efficient way to purify water. Note that iodine is banned for this use in the EU but available elsewhere. Iodine kills most bacteria, viruses, and cysts depending on temperature, concentration, and duration of contact. The addition of 8 mg of iodine per litre of water at 20°C for 10 minutes destroys virtually all pathogens (see question 7).

2. C. The tough cyst of Cryptosporidium is only eliminated by boiling or filtration.

3. A. One minute boiling is sufficient at sea level, but it is not necessary to bring water to the boil in order to kill all pathogens. Even 70–85°C for 1 minute is usually enough. Some non-pathogenic bacterial spores, e.g. Clostridium, survive at 100°C for over 1 minute.

4. B. Adequate heating is the surest way to sterilize water, although the end result may not look or taste very good. Boiling for 1 minute kills virtually all pathogens. Above 2000 m one must boil for 3 minutes (CDC).

UV irradiation may not get to organisms protected by extraneous material or particulate matter while halogenation as a single-step process does not kill all spores and cysts, e.g. cryptosporidia or giardia.

Filtration can miss some viruses. Iodination combined with microfiltration is generally a very good one-step process.

Reverse osmosis is very promising but still expensive.

5. B. Water boils at progressively lower temperatures as one ascends. Despite this, boiling for 1 minute at 3048 m (10,000 feet) probably renders water safe to drink, although not sterile. However, most would boil it for longer to exclude any margin of error.

6. A. Vitamin C combines with free iodine in water and so masks the taste of iodine. Vitamin C should only be added after sufficient contact time between iodine and water has elapsed for disinfection to occur. Other ways of improving taste include adding thiosulfate or hydrogen peroxide.

7. A. Iodine is easier to manage than chlorine although the latter is widely used in large-scale disinfection. Iodine concentrations as low as 0.25 ppm are effectively bactericidal except for mycobacteria (500 times more resistant).

8. A. Proper halogenation is effective against most viruses. Both iodine and chlorine are widely available, easy-to–use, and inexpensive disinfectants for drinking water but all halogens are relatively ineffective in cloudy water. Iodine generally needs 20 minutes of contact with clear water to exert full effects. However, low concentrations of iodine are more persistent and effective than similar concentrations of chlorine. Reports of hyperthyroidism in Peace Corps workers using iodine for protracted periods point to the need to instruct the traveller how to use iodine correctly. However, even with long contact time, either halogen is unlikely to kill all parasitic larvae and protozoal cysts, including those of *Cryptosporidium parvum*, *Giardia lamblia* and probably cyclospora. Filters of 1 µm are used to remove parasitic cysts.

Iodine resin filters contain carbon to remove residual iodine. In 2004 over 1000 laboratory-confirmed cases of giardia occurred in Bergen, Norway due to a contaminated but halogenated unfiltered water supply. UV treatment has since been installed. Although iodine is easier to manage than chlorine, the latter is widely used in large-scale disinfection where a concentration of 0.25 ppm is bactericidal (see question 7).

9. D. It is important to wash dishes according to the sequential three-dish rule. One example is to clean utensils well using detergent in bowl 1, transfer to bowl 2 to which chlorine or bleach is added, and finally rinse in drinking water in bowl 3. Hot water enhances the value of this regime in preventing infectious diarrhoea.

10. D. In an emergency one can drink water to which household bleach (4–6% chlorine) has been added (2 drops/l or 8 drops/gallon). If this is not available one can filter the water through a clean cloth and allow it to settle for 30 minutes. If there are facilities, boil the water.

Apparently clean spring water is often infected with human or animal excreta.

Rafting

1. A. Freshwater drowning is the most common cause of death. It is not possible to state the role of trauma, especially head injury, as a contributory factor.

2. A. Leptospires, which abound in the urine of infected animals, especially rats, can penetrate intact skin, mucus membranes, or conjunctiva. Long immersion, cuts, and abrasions facilitate entry.

3. C. Leptospirosis, most often due to *L. interrogans*, is a worldwide disease except in the polar regions. It is becoming more frequent in travellers who take part in water activities overseas. A history of exposure together with conjunctival suffusion and myalgia are considered pathognomonic, but it is hoped that a quick urine dipstick test, based on leptospira-specific IgM, will displace other more complicated and slower microscopic agglutination tests (MAT tests).

4. C. The incidence of leptospirosis per 100,000 per year is as follows: Seychelles 101, Cuba 2.5, Queensland 2.1, Italy 0.13. Most post-travel cases are acquired in South-East Asia, the Caribbean, and Central and South America. One study in Cambodia showed that leptospirosis accounted for 14% of febrile cases presenting to health centres, which was greater than dengue, malaria, typhoid, or influenza. Leptospirosis is difficult to diagnose and carries up to 30% mortality globally with up to 500,000 cases being reported each year.

Climate extremes

1. A. A breakdown of consultations in Antarctic bases puts injury at around 42%, respiratory illness at 9.7%, skin and subcutaneous problems at 9.6 %, infection and parasitic disease at 7.3%, musculocutaneous and connective tissue problems at 7.1%, and psychiatric disturbance at 2.3%.

2. C. Dental problems greatly outnumber any problems that are specifically associated with the environment.

3. B. Frostbite accounts for up to 95% of cold-related problems in skiers and snowmobilers. Luckily it is mostly superficial.

4. C. Frostbite occurs at temperatures<0°C, especially if clothes or gloves are wet and there is a wind. Frostnip is a much milder form of frostbite. More than 80 cases are admitted to Chamonix hospital in the French Alps each year.

5. C. Adequate fluid intake is vital to prevent dehydration, otherwise water for sweating is provided from the extracellular fluid with subsequent hypotension, a rise in body core temperature, and inevitable heat exhaustion. Light-coloured clothes help by reflecting the sun's rays. Wearing shorts allows extra skin exposure for evaporation of sweat. Overall, however, local humidity is the major controller of the evaporation of sweat and hence of the ability to keep the body cool. Fans are useful cooling devices but depend on factors such as availability, practicality, and the local electricity supply.

6. B. Alcohol slows acclimatization to heat, cold, and altitude. A nearly colourless urine indicates the traveller is drinking sufficient for the body's needs. Humidity slows acclimatization by interfering with perspiration. Some drugs hinder acclimatization, e.g many antihypertensives, anti-Parkinson preparations, antihistamines, and antidepressants.

7. D. Travellers to hot environments are encouraged to drink copiously, at least 4 l/day. However, by drinking inordinate amounts of water, beer, or tea travellers can easily become water intoxicated, with consequent hyponatraemia. This is compounded by the fact that, although sweat is normally hypotonic, it takes 4–7 days before the sodium concentration in sweat falls significantly further (heat acclimatization).

Nausea, vomiting, and headache make hyponatraemia difficult to distinguish from heat exhaustion. As hyponatraemia progresses, convulsions and coma can occur and these signs of cerebral edema must be distinguished from hypoglycemia and hyperthermia.

Acidosis and hypoglycaemia are the results of inordinate exercise in any environment.

8. D. The first priority is to reduce body core temperature. Other priorities can follow. Immersion in ice causes vasoconstriction in skin and subcutaneous tissue. This diverts warm blood from the body shell to the body core and further increases core temperature. The alternate warm/cool exposure devised by Nasr El Din and his colleagues for those doing the Hajj pilgrimage during the hot months of summer overcomes this problem (personal communication).

Snakes and scorpions

1. A. Immobilize the whole affected limb with splints and apply firm but not tight bandaging. This limits the spread of toxin and the amount of local tissue damage. Incisions, suction, and tight compression can all be harmful. Note that thorough washing out of the bite area is required in all cases. Most venomous snakes are especially active at night.

2. C. Elapids cause the greatest number of deaths, usually with severe local myonecrosis and respiratory paralysis. Vipers cause the greatest number of bites with local pain, coagulopathy, and distant organ damage. Scorpions, often hiding in footwear or in one's shower, cause a significant number of deaths worldwide but still fewer than those due to snakes. The vast bulk of arthropod stings are caused by hymenoptera (bees, wasps, ants).

3. C. Between 50% and 70% of people bitten by a venomous snake develop signs of envenomation. These vary from local swelling and necrosis to systemic phenomena such as blood-clotting disorders, CVS abnormalities, rhabdomyolysis, hanematuria, and hypovolaemic shock. Sea snakes are noted for myo- and neurotoxicity.

4. B. Vipers bite readily and can attack without provocation. Most deaths occur in Asia. Overall the elapids are the chief culprits. Bites in children are more dangerous because of their small body mass. Remember the rhyme about coral snakes: 'red on yellow kill a fellow, red on black venom lack'.

5. C. The pain of a spider or scorpion sting is acute and intense. You will notice it! Associated autonomic dysfunction can be life-threatening. This is manifest by lacrymation, sweating, tachypnoea, tachycardia, and abdominal colic followed by pulmonary oedema, cardiac arrhythmias, and either massive hypotension or hypertension. In many places stings from scorpions and spiders are more common than snakebites. Serious cases should be hospitalized.

Marine envenomations and injuries

1. B. Two potentially deadly jellyfish occur in tropical waters, Chirodropids and Iruandji. Acute anaphylaxis, cardiac or respiratory arrest, or massive hypotension can come on in a few minutes. Since the first fatal sting was reported from Australia in 1884 many others have occurred, sometimes in tourists swimming in popular resorts, e.g Pattaya and Koh Samui.

Vinegar denatures the venom of jellyfish and when applied locally is very helpful in easing the pain. Anecdotally the extract from a local Asian plant (*Ipomoea pes-caprae*) appears even better. Sea lice (hydromedusae) cause typical pinpricks and live in conditions similar to those in which box jellyfish thrive. Wearing panty-hose when swimming is said to be effective in preventing jellyfish stings.

2. A. Shockers deliver an electric shock that is rarely a problem unless the victim is already unconscious or aspirates water.

Hot water counteracts the effects of the thermolabile toxins of 'stickers' (lion-scorpion or stone-fish, stingray).

'Scrapers', such as coral, cause direct trauma to the skin and bacterial infection together with envenomation and inflammation follows if fragments of coral are left in the skin.

Jellyfish are classed as 'stingers'.

The fifth type of biological marine injury is caused by 'snappers'. These include sharks and other game fish which cause direct physical trauma.

War zones

1. D. While all the above are important it is vital to have a clear means of identifying oneself as an official non-combatant. Cameras, expensive watches, medicines, and money are all suspect and are often confiscated by patrols. Patience and courtesy are essential elements in making your way through a danger zone. Do not attempt to take a photograph without explicit permission. Sharing liquor or cigarettes, although wrong in principle, is widely expected.

Swimming

Drowning is a hazard for the international traveller whether swimming, snorkeling, scuba diving, or boating. Alcohol always exacerbates the danger. Drowning in children is a particular problem. In one British study (1996–2003) 74% of drowning in children <14 years old occurred in swimming pools.

1. **Which of the statements is true of drowning?**
   A. Drowning is more common in fresh than in salt water
   B. Drowning is faster in sea than in fresh water
   C. Drowning always occurs within the first 12 hours
   D. Drowning is always associated with water entering the small airways and alveoli

2. **Which of the statements is true of childhood drowning?**
   A. Usually children scream and splash when in danger
   B. Rigid pool covers and alarms reduce danger
   C. Four-sided pool fencing reduces the danger
   D. Access to intensive care facilities reduces mortality

3. **A 19-year-old male swimmer has been home for a week after taking part in an international triathlon in Beijing where he spent 10 days. He received all the usual immunizations before leaving the USA and was careful about his diet. He says he was not bitten by anything. He lived in excellent accommodation and took no antimalarials. He now complains of fever, headache, and myalgia, mainly in the calves. On examination he has conjunctival suffusion affecting the palpebral conjunctiva. There is no rash. Which of the following is the most likely?**
   A. Malaria
   B. Dengue fever
   C. Legionnaires' disease
   D. Leptospirosis

4. **Primary amoebic meningoencephalitis (PAM) due to *Naegleria fowleri***
   A. Is acquired by nasal inhalation of water that is contaminated by *N. fowleri*
   B. Is more common after exposure to colder waters (<10°C)
   C. Is mainly acquired by activities in sea (salt) water
   D. Is more likely to occur in adults than in children

Diving

1. **For every 10 m (33 feet) descent in salt water the ambient pressure increases by the equivalent of**
   A. Half an atmospheric pressure
   B. One atmospheric pressure
   C. Two atmospheric pressures
   D. Five atmospheric pressures

2. **You can normally expect a casual swimmer to breath-hold in a 'free' dive for about**
   A. 1–2 minutes
   B. 2–5 minutes
   C. 5–6 minutes
   D. >6 minutes

3. **Hyperventilation before a free dive**
   A. Raises the PaO_2 significantly
   B. Renders the person less susceptible to the narcotic effects of CO_2
   C. Permits the diver to stay submerged longer
   D. Increases cerebral blood flow (CBF)

4. **Diving with self-contained underwater breathing apparatus (SCUBA)**
   A. Allows divers to swim comfortably at depths of 100 m (330 feet)
   B. Allows divers to swim comfortably at depths of 40 m (130 feet)
   C. Involves the use of a tank filled with oxygen
   D. Allows the pressure of inhaled O_2 (PiO_2) approximate to its sea level pressure (155 mmHg)

5. **Barotrauma refers specifically to damage of**
   A. Middle ear ossicles by high altitude
   B. Middle ear ossicles when below sea level
   C. Tympanic membrane when diving
   D. Any air-filled body cavity due to inequality of inside and outside pressures

6. **The risk of barotrauma from diving is most pronounced**
   A. Near the surface
   B. At the greatest depth attainable
   C. At a depth of 99 feet (4 atmospheres)
   D. After completing a dive

7. **For a patient with a history of epilepsy who hopes to scuba dive while on holiday overseas you should**
    A. Tell him to make sure his epilepsy is well controlled before diving
    B. Increase his anti-epilepsy medication for the period over which he plans to dive
    C. Advise him to go ahead but always have a companion nearby when diving
    D. Turn him down completely as a candidate for scuba diving

8. **The most common cause of death in divers is**
    A. Drowning (inhalation of water)
    B. Pulmonary barotrauma
    C. Cardiovascular events
    D. Cerebrovascular accident

9. **Which is the most common part of the body affected by barotrauma?**
    A. The lungs (pulmonary overpressurization syndrome, POPS)
    B. The skin ('mask barotrauma')
    C. The middle ear
    D. The GIT

10. **Barotrauma during ascent from a dive most often occurs in**
    A. The lungs
    B. The middle ear
    C. The face
    D. The paranasal sinuses

Mountain climbing

1. **The Lake Louise criteria for acute mountain sickness (AMS) specifically**
    A. Refer to ascent over 1500 m (5000 feet)
    B. Refer to the level of oxygen in the climber's blood
    C. Name sleep disturbance as the primary symptom of AMS
    D. Name headache as the primary symptom of AMS

2. **In practice the most common initial symptom of AMS is**
    A. Vomiting
    B. Diarrhoea
    C. Headache
    D. Vertigo

3. **In unacclimatized people AMS is most likely to occur in**
   A. Women
   B. Unfit persons
   C. Those with a history of previous attacks of AMS
   D. Those taking alcohol or other depressants

4. **On travelling rapidly from sea level to 2500 m (8000 feet)**
   A. The majority of people have no symptoms at all
   B. The majority of people have mild symptoms
   C. If AMS occurs it will do so almost immediately on arrival at the new high altitude
   D. The likelihood of AMS is the same at the same altitude in Alsaka and in Nepal

5. **What advice should you give if you suspect AMS?**
   A. Take dexamethasone immediately
   B. Start acetazolamide (Diamox™) immediately or increase the dose if the climber is already taking it
   C. Rest at this level until symptoms resolve
   D. Descend immediately

6. **Which of the following is the most efficacious in preventing/treating AMS?**
   A. Acetazolamide
   B. Theophylline
   C. Dexamethasone
   D. Ginkgo biloba

7. **Acetazolamide (Diamox™) is generally recommended**
   A. For a week before and after ascent
   B. Once the climber has reached 2500 m
   C. 24 hours before ascent and 48 hours afterwards
   D. Once symptoms of AMS have started

8. **Adverse reactions of acetazolamide include**
   A. Tingling in the extremities
   B. Insomnia
   C. Urinary retention
   D. Alkalosis

9. **What is the minimum number of persons needed to treat (NNT) at different dosages of acetazolamide for the prevention of AMS compared to placebo?**
   A. Three if on 750 mg per day
   B. Seven if on 500 mg per day
   C. 100 if on 250 mg per day
   D. 200 if on 125 mg per day

10. **Which of the following is an ominous finding in AMS?**
    A. Retinal hemorrhages
    B. Ataxia
    C. Brain swelling
    D. Altered sleep pattern with periodic breathing

11. **A climber complains of headache, fatigue, diarrhoea, anorexia, dry cough, and some incoordination at 3000 m (9000 feet). You must especially consider**
    A. Covert drinking of alcohol
    B. Incipient high-altitude pulmonary oedema (HAPE)
    C. Incipient high-altitude cerebral oedema (HACE)
    D. Early dehydration

12. **Risk factors for HAPE include**
    A. Being an adult rather than a child
    B. Being overheated, e.g. in mufflers and parka
    C. First time rapid ascent
    D. Abnormal response to or faulty production of nitric oxide (NO)

13. **What is the earliest indication of HAPE?**
    A. Breathlessness on exertion
    B. Breathlessness at rest
    C. Pulmonary crackles
    D. Blue lips

14. **The management of HAPE includes**
    A. Diamox
    B. A calcium channel blocker, e.g. nifedipine
    C. Gingko biloba
    D. Dexamethasone

15. **Which of the following is true of HAPE?**
    A. HAPE frequently affects the middle lobe of the right lung
    B. HAPE is less common than HACE
    C. HAPE rarely occurs in children
    D. HAPE is associated with a widespread sudden constriction of pulmonary capillaries

16. **Altitude-induced hypobaric hypoxia causes**
    A. Pulmonary vasoconstriction
    B. Pulmonary vasodilation
    C. Cerebral vasoconstriction
    A. Coronary vasoconstriction

Swimming

1. A. Approximately 75% of drownings occur in fresh water and 25% in the sea. Freshwater drowning can occur in a few minutes. In these cases the blood volume may increase by as much as 50% in 3 minutes due to the osmotic passage of water across the pulmonary alveolar/capillary membrane. Pulmonary oedema occurs in saltwater drowning and death is slower. In both cases hypoxaemia, acidosis, and unconsciousness ensue.

Dry asphyxia occurs in up to 20% of cases, with laryngeal spasm preventing the entry of water into the bronchial tree. Up to 25% of those resuscitated immediately after near-drowning die within 24 hours, so-called 'secondary drowning'.

Drowning is an added danger for the holidaymaker who swims in an unknown or isolated location where currents, alcohol, inexperience, and lack of help become major contributory factors. Drowning is the third most common cause of death in children in the USA after road traffic accidents and burns. *Note*: hypothermia is an important factor in drowning at sea.

2. C. Climb-resistant pool fencing and self-closing gates have been proved to reduce the danger of drowning in children.

Pool covers and alarms are often out of order, usually children drown silently, often when the supervisor is momentarily distracted. Immediate CPR is of help but the outcome is not improved after transfer to an ICU. Neither personal flotation devices nor inflatable life vests appear to reduce the incidence of drowning in those <14 years of age.

3. D. It is said that conjunctival suffusion and myalgia are pathognomonic of Leptospirosis, both of which were present in the above case. Leptospires are highly motile spirochetes harboured in the kidneys of many wild and domestic animals. They are shed continually in the urine. Humans are infected through skin abrasions or mucus membranes contacting infected freshwater. The disease is on the increase and is often reported in travellers who take part in water sports.

Icteric leptospirosis (Weil's disease) occurs in 5–10% of all cases. This has a high mortality if untreated. However, leptospirosis is mostly asymptomatic. Inexplicably it appears to be a milder condition in women.

Malaria is more or less confined to south-west China, especially Hainan, where *P. falciparum* occurs. Otherwise any malaria found is the 'benign form'. Dengue fever is common in China and must be excluded despite the fact that he says he got no bites.

Legionnaire's disease is a possibility but pulmonary symptoms are usually prominent.

4. A. *N. fowleri* is a free-living thermophilic amoeba-type organism found globally in warm fresh waters such as hot springs, spas, untreated swimming pools, ponds, lakes, and sewage. It is found in three forms: as a cyst, as a trophozoite (amoeboid), and as a biflagellate.

The trophozoites thrive between 30 and 46°C and enter the cranium via the cribriform plate. This ensures that the trophozoites are more likely to affect children in whom the cribriform plate is thinner than in adults. When the temperature falls the trophozoites revert to thick-walled cysts, which are still infective as a dust aerosol. These inactive cysts revert to infective trophozoites once the temperature rises again.

PAM has a short incubation period (24 hours to 8 days) and is almost always fatal, although it may respond to amphotericin B with miconazole and rifampin as secondary agents. Although PAM was only described in Australia in 1965 a case may have occurred in Ireland as far back as 1909.

Diving

1. B. One atmospheric pressure on the earth's surface is 760 mmHg or 14.7 psi (pounds/inch²). Pressure increases by this amount for every 10 m descent in salt water (10.30 m in fresh water).

2. A. Breakpoint in breath-holding depends on hypoxia, CO_2 retention, training, and psychological factors. Even the famous Ama pearl divers of Japan seldom remain submerged for over 3–5 minutes. Occasional reports of extraordinary periods of breath-holding under water at remarkable depths have been recorded, e.g. Pippin Ferrera's free dive to 134 m (439 feet) in 1996 when he held his breath for 14 minutes. Peter Colat, a Swiss free diver, held his breath in a water tank for 19 minutes and 21 seconds in 2010.

3. C. Hyperventilation is widely used before a free dive in order to prolong the time submerged. It does this by washing out CO_2 and thus causing a fall in hydrogen ion levels in the CSF. CSF hydrogen ion concentration is the primary stimulus for respiration so that by removing this stimulus the diver can prolong breath-holding significantly.

Unfortunately, because of the consequent lack of the desire to breathe, progressive hypoxemia can occur to such an extent that the subject becomes unconscious.

Hyperventilation does not raise the PaO_2 significantly.

CBF is increased by hypercarbia and hypoxaemia, and is decreased by hypocarbia and hyperoxaemia. CBF is therefore decreased in hyperventilation.

4. B. Scuba diving ('aqualung') was introduced by Jacques Costeau and Emile Gagnan in 1943 and is now used by divers worldwide. It is recommended that one should not go deeper than approximately 40 m for comfort and safety.

The scuba diver's tank contains compressed air, not oxygen, at approximately 200 atmospheres. This is delivered to the diver via a series of reduction valves at around 10 atmospheres (100–160 psi). There is a corresponding increase in the PiO_2.

No one should attempt a scuba dive without having been first fully instructed and supervised.

5. D. Barotrauma occurs because of a failure to equalize inside and outside pressures. It can therefore affect many organs, e.g. the middle ear, the paranasal sinuses, the teeth, the gastrointestinal tract, the lungs, and the face.

6. A. The risk of barotrauma is most pronounced near the surface, where a small change in depth—even a few metres—may lead to a large change in gas volume (Boyle's law: the volume of a gas varies inversely with the pressure provided the temperature remains constant $P_1V_1 = P_2V_2$).

7. D. The danger of convulsions is increased even in normal people in scuba diving. Underwater seizures can be fatal. Those with epilepsy should not be allowed dive and neither should those prone to pneumothorax, asthma, or respiratory tract infection, or those who have had previous chest surgery, have diabetes, or even those with a history of chronic ear disease, especially with scarring of the tympanic membrane.

8. A. Drowning is the most common cause of death in divers followed by pulmonary barotrauma or pulmonary overpressurization syndrome (POPS). In POPS there is overdistension of the lungs and subsequent arterial gas embolism (AGE).

9. C. Middle ear barotrauma accounts for up to 60% of reported cases. The paranasal sinuses are the second most common.

10. A. POPS results from alveolar rupture and can result in pneumomediastinum, pneumothorax, subcutaneous emphysema, or AGE. It is seen most often in scuba divers ascending rapidly from a deep dive. In such a case the lungs re-expand as the diver approaches the sea level but clearly this expansion cannot exceed the original lung volume.

At this point, unless the pent-up high-pressure intraalveolar 'air' can escape via the nose or mouth, there is an imminent danger of alveolar rupture. Breath-holding futher increases the danger during a too rapid ascent.

Damage to the middle ear (cannot open Eustachian tube), face (facial tissue pulled into the mask), and sinuses is most likely during descent.

Mountain climbing

1. D. The Lake Louise Consensus (1991, 1993) states that AMS can occur in unacclimatized people 3–36 hours after a rapid ascent to an altitude >3000 m (>984.2 feet). The following criteria were proposed for AMS: headache worsened by lying down and any one of nausea, fatigue, dizziness, or insomnia. Note that not every case of AMS presents with headache but it is wise to consider AMS in anyone who otherwise fulfils the criteria.

2. C. Most report severe bifrontal headache as the earliest symptom. The headache is worsened by bending over, performing the Valsalva manoeuvre, or lying down. However, fatigue, dyspnoea on exertion, difficulty sleeping, and anorexia are also frequent findings.

3. D. AMS is independent of gender, physical fitness, previous attacks, or even smoking. It is more likely to occur in those >55 years of age, those who are drinking alcohol, taking depressant drugs, e.g. hypnotics, are mildly dehydrated, or are overexerted, e.g. carrying heavy loads. The occurrence of AMS is dependent on the elevation, rate of ascent, and individual susceptibility.

4. A. A height of 2500 m (8000 feet) is considered a safe high altitude for normal people. If symptoms occur they are minimal and confined to very few people, usually to those with pre-existing anaemia or cardiopulmonary disease. AMS generally takes up to 36 hours to develop so there is plenty of time to consider this diagnosis in anyone complaining of headache, insomnia, or undue fatigue.

Because of the shape of the earth someone on the summit of Denali in Alaska is subject to 15–20% greater hypoxia than someone at the same altitude in the Himalayas.

Recall that 75% of people will have mild symptoms at over 3000 m (9000 feet).

5. C. The majority of cases of AMS are benign and self-limiting, and acclimatization occurs if there is no further ascent for 12–36 hours. However, should the climber not improve in that period or should symptoms get worse at any time, immediate descent is imperative.

6. A. All are useful in the prophylaxis and treatment of AMS apart from Ginkgo biloba, which has questionable value. However, acetazolamide is probably the most effective. The doses of each are acetazolamide 500–750 mg/day or 125 mg bid or 500 mg (slow release) SR Q12h, theophylline low dose, 300 mg SR/day, starting 5 days prior to ascent, and dexamethasone 4 mg Q6H.

7. C. Blood levels after oral Diamox peak 1–4 hours after regular and 3–6 hours after SR tablets. Thus starting Diamox 24 hour before ascent and continuing for 48 hours after descent is reasonable, although authorities differ concerning the dosage (see question 6).

8. A. Tingling in the extremities is very common and even the tongue may be involved. Studies on climbers show that sleep patterns are improved and symptoms of AMS are relieved (headache, dizziness, nausea, dyspnoea, fatigue).

Acetazolamide is a carbonic anhydrase inhibitor and therefore it causes diuresis and acidosis due to sodium loss in urine. It is subject to the same adverse reactions as any sulpha drug. Those on high doses may have distortion of normal taste (dysgeusia) and may find a metallic taste from carbonated beverages, perhaps by inhibiting lingual carbonic anhydrase.

9. A. The NNT for acetazolamide according to one meta-analysis is three. This does not mean that lower doses of the drug are without value. All three dosage schemes are better than placebo. It is not clear whether adverse side effects (tingling and polyuria) are significantly greater with the larger doses.

10. B. Ataxia, demonstrated by a failure to do heel/toe walking correctly, is a portent of HACE. Retinal hemorrhages are common and almost always resolve spontaneously with no permanent damage. They are presumably due to hypoxic cerebral vasodilation.

Brain swelling is usually observed in climbers and provided it is not >3ml it is quickly compensated by displacement of CSF.

Altered sleep pattern and periodic breathing are very frequent and are corrected by giving acetazolamide.

11. C. Consider all options, especially HACE. This must be ruled out urgently because the onset of incoordination, especially truncal ataxia, is a potentially very serious sign in a climber. In this case oxygen should be given and the climber brought to a lower altitude immediately, otherwise coma may rapidly supervene.

Both pulmonary and cerebral oedema are serious progressions of AMS and carry a high mortality unless swift action is taken.

Dry air often gives the climber a reactive cough while covert alcohol drinking can easily be checked in a group of climbers.

12. D. HAPE occurs in up to 10% of those who ascend rapidly to 4500 m (14,764 feet). It is six times more common in children than in adults. Risk factors include cold, exercise, previous HAPE, and abnormalities of the NO system.

NO is a powerful endogenous pulmonary vasodilator that counteracts hypoxic pulmonary vasoconstriction, a central feature of HAPE. Vascular endothelium is the major site of NO production in the body.

The incidence of HAPE is about 1.6% in Mount Everest trekkers.

13. B. All of us suffer from breathlessness on exertion but breathlessness at rest is abnormal and is the earliest sign of HAPE. According to the Lake Louise Criteria the diagnosis of HAPE can be made if a person at high altitude has at least two of the following symptoms: chest tightness, markedly decreased exercise performance, dyspnoea at rest, and cough together with any two of central cyanosis, pulmonary crackles, tachycardia >110, and tachypnoea >20.

14. B. SR sublingual nifedipine (20 mg capsule) every 8 hours helps lower pulmonary artery pressures. Sildenafil can also cause pulmonary vasodilation. Diamox is used in AMS while dexamethasone 8 mg IM may be useful in high-altitude cerebral oedema. Note that a portable compression chamber is a most valuable piece of equipment for the emergency relief of any low-pressure syndrome.

15. A. The middle lobe of the right lung is frequently affected in HAPE. This is probably due to the altered dynamics of pulmonary blood flow at high altitude. Capillary permeability is increased but of course capillaries are amuscular and therefore cannot constrict. However, there is uneven constriction and dilation of pulmonary arterioles, which leads to over- and under-perfused regions of the lungs. This constitutes a fundamental problem in HAPE.

HAPE occurs as often in children as in adults and is, overall, more frequent than HACE.

16. A. A fall in PaO_2 causes vasodilation virtually everywhere in the body except in the lungs, where arteriolar constriction occurs.

FISH HAZARDS

Most people know that, apart from choking on a fish bone, eating fish overseas can cause a variety of gastrointestinal upsets. Most travellers would not wish to eat raw fish. However, raw fish dressed up in spices or marinated or undercooked may well be acceptable to them, especially in a foreign land. There are also occasional dangers in eating some fish that are salted or even well-cooked, and which look, smell, and taste normal.

1. **Ciguatera fish poisoning (ciguatoxin, maitotoxin) is**
   A. Most common after eating fish caught in waters off Japan
   B. Less severe after previous exposure to small doses of ciguatoxin or maitotoxin
   C. Associated with enhanced sensitivity to pressure on the skin
   D. Associated with temperature reversal where cold objects feel hot and hot objects feel cold

2. **Ciguatera fish poison**
   A. Is fairly evenly distributed throughout the affected fish
   B. Is most common in small reef fish
   C. Can be identifed using a commercial immunoassay kit
   D. Has only been recorded in humans in recent times

3. **Scombroid fish poisoning**
   A. Is virtually confined to tropical waters
   B. Only becomes symptomatic >48 hours after eating the affected fish
   C. Is due to the presence of histamine in the affected fish
   D. Will only occur if the fish is raw or under-cooked

4. **Which of the following is true for fugu or puffer fish poisoning (tetrodotoxin poisoning)?**
   A. Affected fish sometimes have a peppery taste
   B. Is most common off the Great Barrier Reef
   C. Has an insidious onset over 24–72 hours
   D. Toxin levels are highest in the ovaries of the fish

5. **Match the syndromes in the left-hand column with the toxin options listed on the right. Options may be used once, more than once, or not at all**

    A. Scombroid   1. Tetrodotoxin
    B. Amnesic shellfish poisoning   2. Histamine
    C. Ciguatera   3. Maitotoxin
    D. Fugu (pufferfish)   4. Domoic acid

6. **Which of these shellfish are filter feeders?**

    A. Oysters
    B. Lobsters
    C. Crabs
    D. Shrimps

7. **When stung by an envenomous fish**

    A. If possible immerse the stung part in ice cold water
    B. Vigorously rub the affected part
    C. Apply antihistamine cream locally
    D. Use a regional nerve block to relieve severe pain

8. **The most common danger from eating fish when on holiday is**

    A. Fugu poisoning
    B. Fish bone in throat
    C. Typhoid
    D. Salmonella posioning

1. D. Temperature reversal may occur but is not pathognomonic. Ciguatera poisoning is most common in the South Pacific and Caribbean. Previous exposure renders people susceptible to more severe attacks. In endemic areas it is as common as hepatitis A.

Gastroenteritis followed by CVS abnormalities is typical. Early treatment with IV mannitol may be helpful.

2. C. Excellent commercial kits for the identifcation of toxic fish are available (Cigua-check™, Oceanit Test system, Honolulu). The biological chain is as follows. Toxin-producing dinoflagellates are eaten by herbivorous fish, which in turn are eaten by carnivorous ones. Humans are most likely to eat large carnivorous reef fish such as shark, barracuda, moray eel, and sea bass. The poison is concentrated in the head, gut, roe, and liver of the fish. Note that affected fish look, smell, and taste good but are still poisonous even if well cooked.

Ciguatera poisoning was graphically documented by Captain Cooke on his voyage to the South Pacific in 1774. In 2009 an outbreak occurred in a cargo ship that docked in Hamburg.

3. C. Symptoms generally come on within 60 minutes of eating the affected fish. These vary from tuna to mackerel. Symptoms are typical of excess histamine in the body, e.g. flushing, headache, vomiting, diarrhoea, and urticaria. Antihistamines are an effective cure.

Scrombroid poisoning occurs worldwide from eating fish that have been inadequately frozen or improperly stored and in which large amounts of histamine are formed from histidine by bacterial action. It is irrelevant whether the fish is raw, undercooked, well cooked, well cured, or well salted.

4. D. Tetrodotoxin is a water-soluble neurotoxin that is similar to but 50 times more potent than strychnine on a wt/wt basis. It is concentrated in the ovaries, liver, intestine, and skin of affected puffer fish, ocean sunfish, and porcupine fish found mainly off the coast of Japan.

The fugu experience is related to minute doses of the toxin and consists of euphoria and tingling of the lips and general parasthesiae.

CNS symptoms are proportional to the dose ingested and occur rapidly, usually within minutes of eating fugu. Death from respiratory failure can occur but is unlikely if the patient survives for 6 hours. The fish look and taste normal, and the toxin resists heating, cooling, or salting.

5. Answers: A-2; B-4; C-3; D-1

6. A. Filter-feeders concentrate microorganisms and toxins in their bodies. Gastropod molluscs such as periwinkles and bivalve molluscs (oysters, clams, mussels, cockles, and scallops) concentrate microorganisms and toxins in their gills and intestines, especially those toxins made by dinoflagellates and diatoms.

Crustaceans such as shrimps, crabs, lobsters, scampi, and crayfish are mobile animals with hard shells but are not filter feeders. However, they can be contaminated from polluted or infected water and by inadequate or unhygienic handling.

7. D. Standing on a venomous fish or being stung by the nematocysts of a jellyfish can be excruciatingly painful. Regional nerve blocking or local infiltration with lignocaine can bring immediate relief. Most marine venoms are heat labile and immersing in hot water is often helpful. Rubbing is of little value and may spread venom from unburst nematocysts. Vinegar applied locally prevents discharge of nematocysts. Antihistamine creams have no analgesic value. Systemic envenomation is rare but antivenom is available, e.g. in Australia, and is given IV.

8. B. Hardly needs an explanation.

Most travel overseas is by air, although more and more people today, especially the elderly, are taking cruises. Passenger comfort has declined over the past 40 years despite the advances in aeronautics. This is due to the huge increase in the numbers travelling, the existence of cheaper flights, and the lack of staff to cope with the numbers of passengers both in airports and during flights.There is severe stress associated not only with air travel *per se* but also with all its accompaniments, such as getting through security, checking passports, tickets, and luggage, fear of overweight bags, finding the right gate, delays and cancellation of flights, missing connections, losing baggage, unexpected strikes, queueing interminably on arrival, and paying airport taxes. This list is seemingly endless.

General

1. **The cabin pressure on commercial aircraft during flying is usually adjusted to about**
   A. Barometric pressure at sea level
   B. 500–1000 m (1500–3000 feet)
   C. 1000–1500 m (3000–4500 feet)
   D. 1500–2500 m (5000–8000 feet)

2. **At cruising level in commercial flights the pressure of oxygen in arterial blood (PaO_2) in healthy people is about**
   A. 95 mmHg
   B. 75 mmHg
   C. 55 mmHg
   D. 40 mmHg

3. **At cruising altitudes, with cabin pressure adjusted to 2500 m (8000 feet), gases in the body cavities expand by about**
   A. 5%
   B. 20%
   C. 30%
   D. 50%

4. **A patient has suffered a compound fracture of the tibia and fibula, and is travelling home by air 24 hours afterwards. He has an above-knee plaster cast on his damaged leg. Should you**
    A. Allow him travel provided the leg is kept well elevated
    B. Make sure his plaster is bivalved before travelling
    C. Replace the solid cast with a pneumatic one
    D. Forbid travel for a few days until his leg edema has reduced

Deep venous thrombosis (DVT)

1. **Travellers' thrombosis and venous thromboembolism (VTE)**
    A. Are dependent on the mode of travel
    B. Have a positive association with air travel of longer than 4 hours
    C. Have only been recognized since 2005
    D. Are grossly over-estimated by calf vein ultrasonography

2. **Which of the following is true for lower limb VTE (DVT and PE)?**
    A. Most cases of DVT are asymptomatic
    B. Symptomatic calf DVT is most unlikely to cause PE
    C. Less than 1% of calf DVTs extend proximally
    D. The death rate from acute PE has fallen dramatically in the past 20 years

3. **DVT in healthy air travellers is**
    A. Virtually unknown in young travellers (<25 years old)
    B. Far more common in females than in males
    C. Far more common in those who travel economy rather than business class
    D. More likely in those who wear below-knee graduated compression stockings (GCS) than in those who wear full-length compression ones

4. **Risk factors for air-travel VTE include**
    A. Ethnic origin
    B. Progesterone-only OCs
    C. People who play contact sports
    D. Economy class travel

5. **Which of the following is true of aspirin?**
    A. Asprin is of proved benefit in the prophylaxis of DVT in travellers over 50 years of age on long-haul flights
    B. Asprin is of proved benefit in the prophylaxis of arterial thrombosis at any age
    C. Asprin is the drug of choice in preventing travel-related DVT
    D. Asprin should be started a week before travel for maximum benefit

Air quality

1. **Which of the following is true of modern commercial airlines and cabin air quality?**
   A. All the air that is introduced comes from outside
   B. Approximately half the air that is introduced comes from outside
   C. Any recirculated air in the cabin comes from the cargo bay areas
   D. Taking air in from the outside is more energy efficient than recirculating air from the aircraft itself

2. **Which of the following is true of commercial airlines and cabin air quality?**
   A. It takes about 30 minutes to fully exchange cabin air
   B. Air from galleys and toilets is ducted overboard
   C. Carbon dioxide (CO_2) levels rise appreciably near the galleys after 8 hours
   D. Ozone (O_3) levels rise appreciably after 8 hours

3. **Chemical contamination of cabin air in modern aircraft**
   A. Is a common problem for pilots
   B. Is a more common problem for flight attendants than for pilots
   C. Is probably due to the formaldehyde used in toilet cleaning materials
   D. Is most likely due to aerosolization of oil fumes from the engines

4. **Which of the following is true for commercial airlines and pollutants?**
   A. Modern ventilation filters fail to remove volatile organic compounds
   B. The modern practice of disinfection of the cabin with permethrin effectively eliminates malaria and other disease-carrying arthropods
   C. The levels of contaminants in airline cabins are at least 10 times higher than in a modern city street
   D. Circulating traces of peanut may cause anaphylaxis in sensitized people

5. **Relative humidity**
   A. Falls to around 5% after a 1–2 hour flight
   B. Is lowest in first class
   C. Is a significant factor in flight-related DVT
   D. Is an contributor to total body dehydration in long-haul flights

6. **Transmission of airborne disease on board aircraft**
   A. Has never been proved
   B. Is most likely in crowded short-haul flights
   C. Is more likely when the aircraft is on the ground
   D. Only occurred on one flight in the SARS outbreak

7. **Which of the following is true for CFUs (colony forming units) and modern high-efficiency particle air filtration (HEPA)?**
    A. There are more pathogenic CFUs in a busy airline cabin than in public places on the ground
    B. HEPA in modern aircraft filters all cabin air
    C. HEPA cannot remove viruses
    D. HEPA removes most odours and volatile organic compounds (VOC)

Contraindications

1. **Cardiovascular contraindications to air travel include**
    A. Myocardial infarction (MI) within the past 3 months
    B. Coronary artery bypass graft (CABG) within the past 3 months
    C. Angina within the past month
    D. Poorly controlled chronic congestive heart failure (CCF)

2. **Pulmonary contraindications to air travel include**
    A. Pneumothorax within 3 months
    B. Asymptomatic pleural effusion (moderate size)
    C. PaO_2 less than 70 mmHg
    D. Contagious pulmonary infection

3. **Hypoxic challenge test (HCT) involves inhaling**
    A. 5% oxygen
    B. 15% oxygen
    C. 50% oxygen
    D. 100% oxygen

Miscellaneous

1. **Food poisoning and commercial air travel is**
    A. Most commonly due to E. coli
    B. Most commonly due to Norovirus
    C. Most commonly due to Salmonella spp.
    D. Most commonly due to S. aureus

2. **Ionizing radiation**
    A. Is greatest over the poles
    B. Is greatest over the equator
    C. Is not significant at altitudes below 13,500 m (40,000 feet)
    D. Has been proved to be linked with some cancers in frequent flyers and cabin crews

3. **Which of the these medical events is the most likely to affect a passenger travelling by air?**
   A. A vasovagal attack
   B. A traumatic incident
   C. An acute respiratory problem
   D. A gastrointestinal upset

4. **Which of the following is true regarding the governance of behaviour in commercial flights?**
   A. A doctor, nurse, or paramedic is obliged to give unsolicited free medical assistance to another passenger in a US plane flying over France
   B. A doctor, nurse, or paramedic is obliged to give unsolicited free medical assistance to another passenger in a French plane on the tarmac in the USA
   C. A fee may be charged for medical assistance if such assistance is specifically requested by the sick passenger or aircrew
   D. In a medical emergency one may be legitimately sued for damages when attending a fellow passenger in an area outside one's own special competence, e.g. a public health doctor inserting a chest drain

5. **The annual risk of of being killed in a road traffic accident compared to being killed while flying is about**
   A. 10:1
   B. 1,000:1
   C. 100,000:1
   D. >5,000,000:1

6. **Myths or not?**
   A. Breast implants can burst while on a plane at 40,000 feet
   B. Perineal damage has been recorded while sitting on a lavatory bowl in an aircraft
   C. Commercial aircraft only discharge washroom waste when flying at high altitudes
   D. The South American Blush Spider (*Arachnius gluteus*) is a frequent inhabitant of airplane toilets

Jet lag

1. **Jet lag is primarily due to**
   A. Lack of sleep/fatigue
   B. Disruption of circadian rhythms
   C. Stress
   D. Irregular meals, excess caffeine, and dehydration

2. **What is the most important external signal for maintaining our circadian rhythm?**
    A. Light/darkness cycle
    B. Body temperature
    C. Habit
    D. Knowledge of events, e.g. of changed time

3. **Jet lag is worst**
    A. After eastward travel
    B. After westward travel
    C. In young adults
    D. In teenagers

4. **Taking melatonin in jet lag helps to**
    A. Prevent and/or treat the effects of jet lag
    B. Promote sleep
    C. Promote alertness
    D. Re-establish cortisol rhythm

5. **Which do you consider the best behavioural method for re-establishing regular circadian rhythm?**
    A. Sunlight
    B. Dietary adjustment
    C. Exercise
    D. Engage in social engagements on arrival

AIR TRAVEL

ANSWERS

General

1. D. Regulations require that cabin air pressure in normal operations not fall below that found at 2438 m (8000 feet). Some variation occurs due to turbulence, the type of aircraft, and weather conditions.

2. C. The normal PaO_2 is about 95 mmHg at sea level and cannot reach 100 mmHg because of venous admixture (anatomical shunts). In healthy people a PaO_2 of 55 mmHg is of little consequence since this represents only a 4% fall in the actual amount of oxygen carried in the blood. At a PaO_2 of 55 mmHg the saturation of haemoglobin with oxygen (SaO_2) is 85–91%, which is almost normal. The explanation lies in the affinity of oxygen for haemoglobin, as demonstrated by the oxyhaemoglobin dissociation curve, where a PaO_2 of 55 mmHg lies on the flat part of the curve. However, flying can seriously compromise those with a low starting PaO_2, say 70 mmHg, at sea level. In this case the person is utilizing the steep part of the curve where even a slight fall in PaO_2 results in a large fall in SaO_2. Thus, when flying, those with cardiopulmonary disease may become severely hypoxic.

3. C. There is no discomfort for the healthy traveller apart from some aural discomfort (middle ear air expands) and abdominal cramps (gastrointestinal gas expands). Those with sinusitis or a heavy cold may have difficulty in equalizing pressures.

4. B. Plaster casts applied within 48 h of air travel should be bivalved in order to prevent gas expansion and consequent pain and even circulatory problems. Pneumatic splints should not be used and are forbidden by many airlines. Instillation of water rather than air into medical devices such as splints, catheters, and cuffed endotracheal tubes can avert expansion problems.

Deep venous thrombosis (DVT)

1. B. The first connection between air travel and DVT was made in 1946 when two elderly men got a DVT on a non-stop 14-hour flight from Boston to Venezeula. In one study of almost 60,000 flights >4 hours, the incidence of VTE in the following 4 weeks was 4.0/1000 compared with 1.2/1000 in non-exposed controls. There are many other studies confirming these findings. Unfortunately there is little uniformity in the criteria used or in the method of follow-up in most studies. DVT in proximal veins (popliteal, iliofemoral) is reliably detected by ultrasonography, but this is not so in calf DVT. There are no clear indications that the mode of travel per se influences the incidence of travellers' thrombosis.

2. A. Most cases of DVT are asymptomatic irrespective of their cause. Up to 25% of calf DVTs can extend proximally and 40% of such cases may cause PE. The prognosis for PE remains unchanged for many years.

DVT is most often found in postoperative patients, especially following hip or pelvic surgery.

3. D. Neither gender nor age per se significantly influence the rate of travel-related DVT in healthy individuals (Scurr Study, 2001). The death of Emma Christofferson from air-related VTE after her Heathrow to Sydney flight in 2000 is evidence that young people are also affected. The LONFLIT study (2003) demonstrated the superiority of GCS over full-length hospital hose.

4. C. Obesity, a history of DVT, thrombophilia, cancer, recent trauma operations, tall stature, HRT, taking oestrogen-containing tablets, varicose veins, seated position with knees flexed, and athletes (multiple traumata) have all been implicated in VTE.

The BEST Study (2003) showed no difference in risk between co-morbidity adjusted business and economy class travellers.

5. B. Aspirin has been registered in Germany for the prevention of arterial thrombosis since 1993. In the PEP Study involving 13,356 patients with hip surgery, aspirin reduced the incidence of DVT by 29% and of PE by 43%. However, it has not been incontrovertibly shown to prevent DVT and PE in air travellers, although the American College of Chest Physicians (2012) do recommend it for high-risk persons travelling long haul. Nonetheless many believe that risks from aspirin, e.g. gastrointestinal bleeding, outweigh any putative benefits. If aspirin is taken, it should be started a few days before travel. A report in 2011 from Germany highlighted the inconsistency and diversity of aspirin prescribing by German physicians for air travellers.

Antithrombin agents such as dabigatran may revolutionize the prevention of DVT in travellers (personal opinion). For example Pradaxa™(dabigratan etexilate) achieves maximum concentration within 0.5–2.0h after administration and has a half life of 12–17h. This drug is ideal for most high risk travellers >18 years of age who have good renal function and are not taking specific medicines such St Johns Wort, antifungals, rifampicin, cyclosporine. Rivaroxaban, an anti-Factor Xa agent, may also prove its usefulness in travel-related DVT.

Air quality

1. B. Modern planes use 50–55% recirculated air (compared to 90% recirculation in office buildings). This is mixed with air from outside. Recirculated air is warmer, moister, more controllable, and more energy efficient to use than outside air. Recirculated air comes from the area above the cabin and under the floor and not from the cargo bays.

2. B. All modern aircraft off-duct as much air as possible from galleys and toilets. Air exchange is complete every 3–5 minutes, in contrast to offices and homes where air exchange occurs every 5–12 minutes. CO_2 levels rise only minimally and most of the ozone (taken in from outside) is converted back to oxygen by the heat of the engines and by catalytic converters.

3. D. There is contamination of cabin air in some older aircraft by vaporized oils from engine cooler systems. This has been associated with a variety of symptoms from dizziness to nausea to overt neurological or autonomic dysfunction. It is likely that no long-term effects occur from such exposure in any group (pilots, attendants, passengers). Nonetheless airline pilots set up the Aerotoxic Association in 2007 to highlight their concerns about this matter.

4. D. Because of this peanuts should no longer be served by airlines. Currently insecticides are applied in a haphazard fashion and almost certainly in amounts that will not kill the growing list of arthropods that are found in aircraft. Airlines will have to review this policy because of the real danger of transferring arthropod-borne disease from one country to another. Filters in older planes do not remove volatile organic compounds and any leak of engine oil or lubricant such as tri-ortho-cresylphosphate (TOCP) can be toxic, in particular to the CNS.

5. B. Relative humidity is lowest where there are fewest passengers per unit area and thus may fall to around 10% in first class and to 20–30% in economy class. Apart from dryness of mucus membranes (eyes, mouth), which may cause some discomfort, the fall in relative humidity is without clinical significance except in those with reactive airways.

Studies have shown that total body water increases in long-haul flights and since much of this may occur in dependent parts, it is theoretically possible that a reduction in cardiac preload may cause a fall in cardiac output in elderly or diabetic people due to impairment of the baroreceptor reflexes.

Dehydration is not a significant factor in causing VTE in airline passengers.

6. C. Environmental control systems (ECS), which remove cabin air, may be switched off while the aircraft is on the ground, thus increasing the risk of disease transmission. As in other situations where people are congregated together, most communicable diseases are transmitted via contact or droplet infection from open cases of infectious disease in persons sitting near the 'victim'. Very few cases of transmission of serious disease have been authenticated in air travellers but in the SARS outbreak of 2003 analysis showed that transmission occurred on five flights involving 29 secondary cases (24 cases on one flight). Disease transmission is far more likely in long-haul flights (time of exposure increased).

7. D. Pall aerospace and Airbus Industrie have now introduced a HEPA/odour/VOC cabin air filter element. Filter efficiency decreases as contaminants accumulate and therefore such filters must be replaced regularly. Modern filters remove particles down to 0.1 μm and are extremely effective in removing moulds, bacteria, and viruses (0.01–0.2 μm). It is not yet possible to pass compressed outside air through modern filters.

Any person-to-person disease transmission in the cabin is usually confined to a couple of seat rows ahead and behind. In this way there have been reports of the transmission of SARS, TB, influenza, and the common cold. There is much concern nowadays at the danger of transmitting MDRTB. See WHO Guidance on TB and Air Travel.

Contraindications

1. D. Uncontrolled or poorly compensated CCF or any uncontrolled arrhythmia are definite contraindications to air travel. So are recent MI or CABG (within 2–3 weeks) and unstable angina. Successful coronary stenting does not appear to be a contraindication after 1–2 weeks.

2. D. A contagious pulmonary condition is always regarded as a contraindication. Anyone with infectious TB must not travel until at least 2 weeks after adequate treatment has started and those with MDRTB must be proved culture negative (WHO, 2006). Pneumothorax within 3 weeks is a definite contraindication to flying and one is better to wait for 6 weeks at least. A large pleural effusion is always a contraindication to flying but small ones are probably safe.

Those with a PaO_2 < 50 mmHg can fly if they order supplemental oxygen from the airline at least 48 hours in advance of their journey. The British Thoracic Society (September 2011) recommend supplemental oxygen if PaO_2 < 50 mmHg (<6.6kPa). They also recommend supplemental oxygen on British Airways commercial flights if the person is taking >4 l/minute oxygen at sea level.

3. B. Hypoxic challenge at a PiO_2 of 15% for 20 minutes is the best single simple test for simulating conditions aboard a commercial airplane and is very useful in deciding how to advise travellers with cardiopulmonary disease. The patient's ability to walk 50 m or climb an average flight of stairs without distress is often used as a yardstick in this regard but has little scientific merit to recommend it.

Miscellaneous

1. C. *Salmonella* spp. can multiply >200 times in 4 hours when taken out of the fridge. This probably accounts for it being the most common cause of poisoning in the airline industry since 1947. This is despite far greater contamination of tested cold airline meals by *S. aureus* and *E. coli* (up to 24%). One breakdown shows the causes of airline gastroenteritis as follows: *Salmonella* spp. 40%, *S. aureus* 19%, *Vibrio* spp. 16% and *Shigella* 9%. Poor temperature storage facilities and contamination by unhygenic food-handlers are the two most important causes. Cold plates, economy class, long-haul flights, and sourcing of meals from hot countries are also implicated in causing this problem.

Note that one study of Royal Air Force (UK) crews showed gastroenteritis was far less common than might be expected. When it did occur many cases were traced to eating contaminated food in the canteen before take off.

2. A. Ionizing cosmic radiation is greatest over the poles and least over the equator. There is no credible evidence linking cancers such as leukaemia with exposure of cabin crew or frequent flyers to cosmic radiation. However, the International Commission for Radiological Protection recommends a maximum exposure dose of 1 milliSievert/year, which is itself an extremely low value. Those who cross the Atlantic more than 10 times a year or fly to Australia more than five times a year probably reach or exceed this limit.

A rough guide is to limit flying to 2000 hours per annum (200 hours if pregnant).

3. A. According to reported incidents compiled by airlines the most common medical events in passengers are vasovagal attack 22%, cardiac 20%, gastrointestinal, respiratory and traumatic each 15%, and others, e.g. cerebrovasccular accident (CVA), hysteria, 8%. Some surveys give different percentages but present a similar stratification of incidents.

4. D. You can be legitimately sued for performing procedures for which you are clearly not trained. The law of the land where the plane is registered is in force when airborne. When on the ground, it is the law of that country which takes precedence. In the USA the Good Samaritan law governs one's actions but no payment is allowed and in many countries, e.g. the UK, medical insurance covers such acts even for non-emergencies, provided there is no payment.

In some countries, e.g. France, it is mandatory to render assistance to a fellow passenger or crew member if asked in an emergency. Neither the patient nor the carrier is legally required to pay for medical services in an air emergency.

5. D. Statistics are confusing, contradictory, and confounded by age, sex, flying frequency, airlines involved, time of year, length of flight, driving habits etc. However, all agree that the risk of death from flying is far less than from a road traffic accident.

6. B. Perineal damage has been authenticated in obese persons using vacuum-flush toilet bowls on commercial flights. It would appear that an airtight seal should be formed between the buttocks and the toilet rim for this to occur. Occasionally it has required outside assistance to separate a passenger from the toilet seat. Vacuum flushing in toilets and wash basins was first introduced by Boeing and is now the norm. All sewage is collected in containers and disposed of later. Breast implants may expand a little but unless there is a serious fault in design the implant will not burst or explode.

Jet lag

1. B. Failure of the body to adapt quickly to a sudden change in time is the cause of jet lag. It usually occurs when six or more time zones are crossed rapidly. Cumulative sleep loss and travel-associated stress and disruption are contributory factors. Symptoms, which often do not come on until the second night after arrival, consist of inappropriate sleepiness and waking, with headache, fatigue, irritability, and poor general functioning also being common.

2. A. Light is the strongest cue but the other options are significant too. External Zeitgebers interact with internal Zeitgebers. The latter primarily maintain the normal diurnal rhythm of the internal milieu, e.g. serum electrolytes, plasma cortisol, plasma renin, vascular tone, and mood.

3. A. Most studies show that jet lag is more pronounced after eastward than westward travel. This is because we can adjust better to a longer than to a shorter day. Jet lag is also more of a problem as one gets older.

4. A. Melatonin has been used since 1986 in the prevention/treatment of jet lag, after Arendt et al. reported on its use in 17 subjects flying from San Francisco to London (eight east time zones). Melatonin undoubtedly helps re-set the 24 hour hypothalamic clock. It also helps lower body temperature and is a mild sedative. Typical doses are 3–5 mg at the new bedtime for 5 days. Melatonin is available OTC in the USA but not in most other countries. Endogenous melatonin from the pineal gland is only secreted at night. There is a suggestion that low-dose sildenafil may be of some use. It undoubtedly is in hamsters (Nature, 2007).

5. A. Exposure to sunlight on arrival (or the use of phototherapy) has been shown to be quite helpful in readjusting circadian rhythms back to normal. Dietary changes help too, but are difficult, involving high and low total calorific intake on alternate days before and after arrival and high-carbohydrate breakfast and lunch for some days after arrival. Pushing oneself into work or social engagements and scheduling oneself to the new time demands is always helpful. Exercise may be of value but not everyone can engage in it.

MEDICAL CARE OVERSEAS

QUESTIONS

One is never really prepared for a mishap or an illness overseas, and whenever such an eventuality occurs one is faced with the problem of accessing the best local treatment. The travel health provider at home should always advise the traveller about the need to check out travel insurance and local medical facilities in the destination before travel, especially in the case of long-term or high-risk travellers.

In addition, the traveller should be given a contact number for the clinic in his or her home country and be instructed to use this contact whenever necessary.

Accessibility and quality

1. **When choosing a doctor overseas**
   A. Be informed before you travel
   B. Use the hotel doctor (assuming a 4-star or better hotel)
   C. Check with another traveller who has experience in that country
   D. Check with local expatriates (embassy, international school, airlines)

2. **When using health services overseas**
   A. If possible choose a doctor who has had experience in your home country
   B. Be pro-active and ask for precise information as often as possible
   C. Establish a doctor–patient relationship
   D. Establish your financial credibility early

3. **When deciding to stay with or leave local care**
   A. Decide as early as possible
   B. Base the decision on the advice of friends
   C. Take note of obvious immediate deficiencies in standards
   D. Leave a definite possibility for your return to that unit

Medical evacuation

1. **When advising travellers on the most appropriate Medivac providers**
   A. Refer them to a health/medical broker
   B. A good list can be found in *Yellow Pages* or its equivalent
   C. Refer to a standard textbook on travel medicine
   D. Tell them to seek information when overseas

2. **Requests for Medivac show that**
   A. The vast majority are urgent problems
   B. The vast majority relate to cardiac problems
   C. The most urgent cases involve the elderly
   D. The need is greatest in travellers who fall ill in sub-Saharan Africa

3. **Which of the following is a criterion for immediate aeromedical evacuation to a facility elsewhere?**
   A. Telephone advice from local physician
   B. Age of patient
   C. Request from immediate relatives at home
   D. Consultation with colleagues at home

4. **Which of the following is an indication for aeromedical evacuation in critically ill patients?**
   A. Bowel obstruction
   B. Ruptured lung cyst
   C. Fulminant hepatitis
   D. Pneumoencephalon

Accessibility and quality

1. A. This is the ideal but not practical unless travelling with a well-established group, e.g. Peace Corps, MSF, VSO, or Oxfam. Checking with a local expatriate is the next best option. Sometimes hotel doctors are excellent, sometimes they are not, and may even share a 'finders fee' with the hotel. Advice from fellow travellers in a hostel, in the bush, or in a local hostelry is notoriously inaccurate.

2. D. It is important for the sick traveller or those with him to clarify financial issues as early as possible. This means checking the traveller's own insurance as well as checking with the healthcare provider.

Sometimes a doctor who has 'experience' in your country may only have done a research project and have little understanding of one's real needs.

Being very pro-active or endeavouring to form a doctor–patient partnership may be interpreted as a challenge and antagonize care providers.

3. D. Always have an exit strategy so that you can leave but return again if necessary. Citing family reasons, insurance reasons, or the need to fulfil obligations at home may allow you leave without damaging relations with the local overseas healthcare provider. You may well need to do this if you know your treatment is sub-optimal.

Many doctors—all over the world—resent being 'corrected' by their patients, so this must be done with tact and courtesy. Immediate surroundings are no guide to the efficacy of care. The well-meaning advice of friends is often impetuous and ill-conceived, and may further bewilder you. A too-early decision is as bad as a too-late decision.

Medical evacuation

1. A. Health/medical brokers have no 'axe to grind' and have access to up-to-date information on appropriate healthcare providers. *Yellow Pages* or travel medicine books are unsatisfactory and often give incorrect contact numbers. Information sought overseas is sometimes marred by local interests.

The discerning traveller can access good information on Medivac providers on the internet. Air-ambulance services via the Marco Polo programme are especially easy to access.

2. D. Analysis of requests for Medivac shows that >75% are non-urgent and most come from travellers in sub-Saharan Africa. The dearth of modern facilities and the frequency of disease in this region probably account for this. Local paediatric facilities are often unsatisfactory in developing countries and so the majority of really urgent requests involve <15-year-olds.

A study from Cologne, Germany, by Sand et al. (2010), showed that the top three diagnoses in 504 adults needing aeromedical evacuation were fracture of the femoral neck (n = 74, 15%), stroke (n = 69, 14%), and myocardial infarction (n = 39, 8%).

A French and also a British study (in diplomats) showed that neuropsychiatric problems account for 15–20% of medical evacuations.

3. B. All of the above may be involved in making the decision to evacuate a patient. The clarity of the diagnosis, the patient's age (especially children), your knowledge of local resouces, the location of the patient, and consultation with colleagues at home and overseas, as well as the wishes of the family, must inform this decision. Children have priority, not only because they cannot make the decision themselves, but because of the lack of paediatric facilities in poorer countries.

In many cases it is important to stabilize the patient as far as possible before transfer. In all cases transfer to the nearest properly equipped hospital—not necessarily to a hospital thousands of miles from the patient's homeland—should be considered, e.g. to South Africa from rural Zambia.

A standard scoring system based on the above would be of great value in making such an important decision.

4. C. Fulminant liver disease, sometimes needing liver transplant, may need urgent transfer to a centre of excellence. The other options are unsafe to transport by air because of the danger of barotrauma.

The next two chapters deal with specific and general medical risks for the traveller. The topics covered are not exhaustive nor are they always exclusive to the traveller. However, they do focus on the problems most likely to be encountered when travelling and, as such, the responsible travel health advisor must be familiar with them.

Travellers' diarrhoea

1. **Acute TD is most likely due to**
   A. *E. coli*
   B. Shigella
   C. Salmonella
   D. Campylobacter

2. **Acute TD**
   A. Can be associated with the Guillian Barré syndrome
   B. Can cause haemolytic uremic syndrome (HUS)
   C. May be associated with the onset of Reiter's syndrome
   D. All of the above are true

3. **Bloody diarrhoea (dysentery) suggests the presence of**
   A. Shigella
   B. Campylobacter
   C. *V. cholera*
   D. Cyclospora

4. **The likelihood of HUS is greatest in diarrhoea because of**
   A. *E. histolytica*
   B. Norovirus
   C. Campylobacter
   D. Specific types of *E. coli*

5. **Humans are the ony natural reservoir for which of the following salmonella species?**
   A. *S. enteretidis*
   B. *S. typhi*
   C. *S. paratyphi* C
   D. *S. dublin*

6. **The most frequent health problem reported during annual military training in Thailand is**
   A. Diarrhoea
   B. Respiratory infections
   C. Sexually transmitted disease
   D. Sunburn

7. **The percentage of Campylobacter isolates resistant to fluoroquinolones (FQ) in the above question is approximately**
   A. 10–20%
   B. 50–80%
   C. 80–90%
   D. >90%

8. **The cause of TD in South-East Asia is now mainly**
   A. *E. coli*
   B. *Campylobacter* spp.
   C. *Vibrio* spp.
   D. Rotavirus

9. **Regarding Campylobacter**
   A. Fewer than 10 organisms can cause TD
   B. Campylobacter organisms are sensitive to gastric HCl
   C. Infective process is strictly confined to the GIT
   D. Transmission is most common by the person-to-person route

10. **TD that lasts more than 1 month is probably due to**
    A. Prolonged bacterial infection
    B. Protozoal infection
    C. Helminths
    D. Unmasking of chronic bowel disease

11. **Regarding cholera and TD**
    A. Cholera causes massive inflammation of gut mucosa
    B. Most cases of cholera cause severe diarrhoea
    C. Ingestion of >10 CFUs is required to cause clinical disease
    D. The biotype 0139 has resulted in several pandemics

12. Comparing cholera and ETEC

A. Both attach to the villi of the small intestine

B. Cholera differs from ETEC in that it also attaches to the mucosa of the large gut

C. The A toxin of cholera is similar to the enterotoxin of ETEC

D. Both cause a secretory diarrhoea by inhibiting cAMP in the intestinal mucosa

13. Persistent diarrhoea after single or multiple antibiotic treatments for TD (including fluoroquinolones, azithromycin, and metronidazole) makes one suspect

A. *Clostridium difficile*

B. Underlying chronic bowel disease, e.g. ulcerative colitis or Crohn's disease

C. Irritable bowel syndrome

D. Amoebic dysentery

14. *C. difficile* is

A. A spirochete

B. A spore-forming fungus

C. Present significantly in the gut flora of most adults

D. Contagious

15. Which of the following is most likely to cause anorexia, abdominal bloating, cramps, flatulence, and watery diarrhoea?

A. *Dientamoeba fragilis*

B. *Giardia lamblia*

C. *Blastocystis hominis*

D. *Entamoeba histolytica*

16. The main reservoir for *Giardia lamblia* is

A. Humans

B. Cats

C. Dogs

D. Farm animals

17. Travellers' Diarrhoea due to *Aeromonas* spp.

A. Is typically blood stained

B. Is the most common cause of TD in Mexico

C. Can cause persistent diarrhoea in travellers

D. Is sensitive to ampicillin

18. *Dientamoeba fragilis*

A. Is an extremely rare cause of TD

B. Is confined to humans

C. Can survive for many months when excreted in the faeces

D. Commonly causes asymptomatic colonization in affected adults

19. The risk of TD is greatest in which of these countries?

    A. Mexico

    B. Thailand

    C. Turkey

    D. Nepal

20. Which of the following organisms is the most likely cause of TD in Bangkok after dining only in top-class restaurants?

    A. *Arcobacter butzleri*

    B. *Campylobacter* spp.

    C. *Salmonella* spp.

    D. *Borrelia* spp.

21. Oral rehydration solution (ORS)

    A. If given properly reduces the frequency of diarrhoea

    B. Should always be hypertonic

    C. Can incorporate rice instead of glucose

    D. Contains NaCl and KCl in equal amounts

22. Blood group A is associated with diarrhoea due to

    A. *Vibrio cholerae*

    B. *Giardia lamblia*

    C. Enterotoxigenic *E. coli* (ETEC)

    D. *Shigella* spp.

23. Diarrhoea is likely once a healthy adult ingests an inoculum of

    A. 100–1000 *V. cholerae* organisms

    B. 100–1000 *E. coli* organisms

    C. 100–1000 *E. histolytica* cysts

    D. 1–100 *G. lamblia* cysts

Prevention of TD

1. Which of the following is your first choice in preventing TD?

    A. Bismuth subsalicylate

    B. An antibiotic

    C. Eat in clean-looking restaurants

    D. Probiotics

SPECIFIC MEDICAL RISKS FOR THE TRAVELLER | QUESTIONS

2. **Adhering to the WHO recommendations concerning food and drink results in**

   A. A significant decrease in TD irrespective of length of travel
   B. A significant decrease in TD in trips <6 weeks in duration
   C. A moderate decrease in TD in most cases
   D. No significant difference

3. **Which of the following is true regarding hand-washing and the spread of disease?**

   A. About 60–70% of people use the soap provided in a rest room
   B. About 60–70% of people wash their hands for more than 10 seconds
   C. Most microorganisms remain long enough on the hands to allow autoinoculation
   D. One is more likely to pick up microorganisms from a clean dry cotton towel than from a door handle

Probiotics, prebiotics, and TD

1. **Which of the following is an accurate definition of probiotics?**

   A. Probiotics are antibiotics in an inactivated form
   B. Probiotics are antibiotics in precursor form
   C. Probiotics are living symbiotic bacteria from animal or human intestine
   D. Probiotics are inactivated symbiotic bacteria from animal or human intestine

2. **Which of the following statements is true of probiotics?**

   A. Probiotics are useful in protecting the traveller against common upper respiratory infections (URIs)
   B. Probiotics are useful in protecting against viral TD
   C. Probiotics sometimes worsen TD
   D. Probiotics are only available on prescription in developing countries

3. **Which of the following statements is true of prebiotics?**

   A. Prebiotics are products of protein digestion
   B. Prebiotics are non-digestible oligosaccharides
   C. Prebiotics were identified and named over 100 years ago
   D. Prebiotics are destroyed during the cooking of food

Skin infestations and infections

1. **Cutaneous leishmaniasis (CL)**
   A. Is transmitted by close contact with someone who already has CL
   B. Is transmitted mainly by the triatomine bug ('kissing bug')
   C. Presents in a similar way wherever it is acquired
   D. May demonstrate 'seeding' at sites of skin trauma or tattoos (Koebner phenomenon**)**

2. **Which of the following is true regarding CL?**
   A. The drug susceptibility of CL correlates with the species of Leishmania
   B. In the Middle East CL typically proceeds to mucocutaneous leishmaniasis (ML)
   C. The Leishmanin test (Montenegro test) is rarely positive in CL
   D. Old World CL (OWCL) rarely heals spontaneously

3. **A major diagnostic help in CL is**
   A. Profound eosinophilia
   B. A positive Leishmanin test
   C. A progressive painless ulcer in someone who has returned from an endemic area
   D. A history of being bitten by insects in an endemic area

4. **Which of the following is true for *Tunga penetrans* (tungiasis, chigoe flea, jigger flea)?**
   A. Males feed intermittently on warm-blooded hosts
   B. Humans are the sole host
   C. It invades subcutaneous tissues
   D. It thrives best in warm humid soil

5. **Which of the following is true for *Tunga penetrans* (tungiasis, chigoe flea, jigger flea)?**
   A. It is an excellent jumper
   B. It can penetrate light shoes, e.g. training shoes
   C. It is more common in adults than in children
   D. It has a life cycle of about 3–4 weeks

6. **Cutaneous myiasis can arise from penetration of the skin by**
   A. Eggs of specific mosquitoes
   B. Eggs of specific flies
   C. Larvae of specific flies
   D. Adults of specific mites

7. **Which of the following is true for African and American cutaneous myiasis?**
   A. Both African and American myiasis are best treated with ivermectin
   B. African myiasis is most likely to occur on exposed places, e.g. head and neck, arms
   C. American myiasis is most likely to be acquired by using non-ironed bed linen and clothing hung outdoors to dry
   D. The little dark head that the examiner sees consists of respiratory spiracles

8. **An itchy moving linear or serpentine lesion under the skin in a patient 7 days back from South-East Asia is most likely to be**
   A. *Cutaneous larva migrans* (CLM)
   B. *Larva currens*
   C. Gnathosyomiasis
   D. Calabar swelling

Moving subcutaneous skin lesions

There are several tropically acquired parasitic skin lesions in which some stage of the parsite's life cycle presents as a migrating subcutaneous lesion. This is usually of a transitory nature. Such stages are characterized by a local allergic inflammatory reaction, pruritus, and eosinophilia. Two of those presented are non-moving although one of them resembles the rest in other respects, e.g. pruritus, local changes in skin pigmentation, local inflammation, and eosinophilia. You are invited to identify these two odd men out.

1. **What is the underlying cause of the subcutaneous lesions observed in each of the following? Options may be used once, more than once, or not at all**

   A. CLM
   B. Bot fly myiasis
   C. Tumbu fly myiasis
   D. Tungiasis (chiggers)
   E. Gnathosyomiasis[b]
   F. Calabar swelling
   G. Onchocercal nodules
   H. Strongyloides[d]

   1. Adult diptera fly
   2. Larva of onchocercal worm
   3. Adult worm (*T. canis* and *T. catis*[a])
   4. Adult non-pregnant female sand flea
   5. Migrating larval worms
   6. Migrating adult loa loa[c]
   7. Adult onchocercal worms
   8. Gravid female sand flea
   9. Larvae of animal hookworms
   10. Larvae of diptera flies

Malaria

1. **The most common factor associated with fatality from imported malaria is**
   A. Incorrect chemoprophylaxis
   B. Failure to diagnose malaria on first visit to doctor/clinic
   C. Failure of the laboratory to identify malaria
   D. Poor choice of drug or route of administration of drug in diagnosed cases

2. **Recurrent attacks of malaria in the traveller are most often due to**
   A. Inadequate treatment of a first attack
   B. Persistent subclinical *P. falciparum*
   C. Persistent subclinical *P. malariae* or *P. knowlesi*
   D. Persistence of the hepatic phase of *P. vivax* or *P. ovale*

3. **Malaria is most likely to present in a traveller coming from an endemic area when the time from exposure to symptoms (ES) is**
   A. 2–6 days
   B. 6–30 days
   C. 1–6 months
   D. 6–12 months

4. **Which of the following is true for 'immunity' to malaria in immigrants from malaria endemic countries?**
   A. It is lost after 1–2 years living in a malaria-free area
   B. It can be demonstrated at least 15 years after leaving a malaria area
   C. Malaria causes a similar duration of fever in non-immune and 'semi-immune' subjects
   D. Malaria has a similar parasite clearance time after treatment in non-immune and 'semi-immune' subjects

5. **Splenic rupture**
   A. Is more frequent in *P. vivax* than in *P. falciparum* malaria
   B. Occurs about equally in *P. vivax* and *P. falciparum* malaria
   C. Should be treated by splenectomy if the rupture is due to malaria
   D. Is almost always associated with a palpable splenic enlargement

6. **Which of the following suggests malaria when the clinical probability of malaria is high?**
   A. Enlarged spleen
   B. Eosinophilia > 500 mm^3
   C. Hb < 14 g/dl
   D. A platelet count < 250×10^9/l

7. **Results from malaria tests (both smear and antigen tests) should be available within**
    A. 3 hours
    B. 12 hours
    C. 24 hours
    D. 48 hours

Rapid diagnostic tests (RDTs)

1. **Which of the following is true for RDTs and malaria?**
    A. RDTs use parasite-specific antibodies to detect malarial antigens in the patient's blood
    B. RDTs use parasite-specific antigens to detect antibodies in the patient's plasma
    C. Results from most RDTs can be read after approximately 30 minutes
    D. RDTs can be used to assess parasite clearance after treating malaria

2. **What is the main problem for the traveller who uses an RDT?**
    A. Placing the blood droplet on the kit
    B. Drawing blood
    C. Waiting the recommended time before reading it
    D. Interpretation of results

3. **Which of the following is correct in regard to malaria RDTs?**
    A. Any lay person can perform the test
    B. They can identify a life-threatening *P. falciparum* infection
    C. Repeat tests are unnecessary
    D. Cost is a major obstacle

Retrospective diagnosis of malaria

1. **Regarding retrospective diagnosis of malaria, which test is best?**
    A. Urine antigen testing
    B. Indirect immunofluorescence antibody test (IFAT)
    C. Blood microscopy
    D. Bone marrow microscopy

Filariasis

1. **Lymphatic filariasis (LF) may be contracted by being exposed to**
   A. Sandflies
   B. Infected body fluids
   C. Soft ticks
   D. Mosquitoes

2. **LF in the traveller and expatriate**
   A. Is almost always asymptomatic
   B. Is associated with microflaraemia shortly after being bitten
   C. Often presents with acute lymphadenitis and lymphangitis
   D. Is curable if Ivermectin is given early in the course of the disease

3. **LF in travellers is usually diagnosed by**
   A. A marked eosinophilia
   B. Finding filarial larvae in the blood
   C. Finding microfilariae in the blood
   D. Immunochromatography (ICT)

Sexually transmitted infections (STIs)

1. **What percentage of Western tourists visiting developing countries admit to having had at least one full sexual contact while on holiday?**
   A. 0.1%
   B. 1.0%
   C. 5.0%
   D. 20.0%

2. **Which of the following is most likely to be contracted after unprotected sex with an unknown partner in a tropical holiday resort?**
   A. Candidiasis
   B. HIV1 or HIV2
   C. Hepatitis B
   D. Syphilis

3. **The percentage rate for syphilis in prostitutes in many developing countries is approximately**
   A. 1.0%
   B. 5.0%
   C. 10.0%
   D. >50.0%

4. **The percentage rate for HIV+ prostitutes in many developing countries can be as high as**

   A. 80%
   B. 50%
   C. 20%
   D. 10%

5. **A female traveller has had casual sex with a local in Uganda. At the time she was menstruating. She says her partner used a condom. She takes oral contraceptives on an irregular basis. What is the most serious problem that faces her?**

   A. Unwanted pregnancy
   B. Gonorrhoea
   C. HIV
   D. *Lymphogranuloma venereum*

6. **Which of the following is a priority for the above patient?**

   A. Use a vaginal douche of soap and water immediately after intercourse
   B. Go on highly active anti-retroviral treatment (HAART) immediately
   C. Taken the 'morning after pill', e.g. levonorgestrel 750 µg (Levonelle™), two tablets up to 72 hours post coitus
   D. Use an antibiotic-containing vaginal gel at least twice a day for 1 week afterwards

7. **Which is the most common opportunistic infection in HIV+ patients?**

   A. *Pneumocystis jirovecii* (formerly *P. carinii*)
   B. Vaginal candidiasis
   C. Pneumococcal infection
   D. Toxoplasmosis

Motion sickness

1. **Which of these behavioural strategies is useful in preventing motion sickness?**

   A. Pressure on the wrist crease
   B. Sitting at mid-point in a bus
   C. Self-controlled regular gentle breathing
   D. Fix eyes on a near object

2. **Motion sickness is less likely to occur in**

   A. Pregnancy
   B. Children under 2 years old
   C. Aerobically trained persons
   D. Men rather than in women

Travellers' diarrhoea

1. A. Enterotoxigenic *E. coli* (ETEC) includes local and diffusely enteroadherent *E. coli* (DEAC) and less frequently the enteroinvasive (EIEC) and enterohaemorrhagic (EHEC) varieties. These account for about 60% of all TDs worldwide. Polymerase chain reaction (PCR) tests have proved that ETEC and DEEC were present in a high number of diarrhoeal stools in cases where the pathogen was classifed as 'unknown'. The acronymn EPEC refers to all enteropathogenic *E. coli*.

2. D. Acute TD is virtually always a benign self-limiting condition in previously healthy people. Nonetheless it may be associated with the serious consequences listed in the question, particularly in elderly, sick, malnourished, or poorly immunogenic individuals. Enteroinvasive and cytotoxic enteropathogens can also cause haemorrhage, bowel perforation, and widespread dissemination. Reiter's syndrome (reactive oligoarthritis [ReA], conjunctivitis, urerthritis/balanitis) can be triggered by many gastrointestinal or genitourinary infections. It has been reported in 7% of cases following *Campylobacter enteritis* and a disquieting 29% of cases following *Salmonella enteritis*, both common causes of TD. ReA can persist for many years.

There is a strong possibility that Christopher Columbus suffered from Reiter's syndrome after a bout of TD. Controversy has arisen concerning the naming of the disease because of Hans Reiter's original misconception about its aetiology and his association with the Nazi party during World War II. It is easy to be put in mind of Reiter's syndrome if one remembers the phrase 'can't see, can't pee, can't climb'.

3. A. Dysentery is typical of shigellosis. However, you must also consider *E. coli* O157, *E.coli* O104, and amoebic dysentery. Occasionally bloody stools occur in malaria and in viral haemorrhagic fevers.

4. D. Shiga-toxin-producing *E.coli* (STEC) can cause HUS in up to 20% of patients (European Centre for Disease Control, ECDC). The outbreaks in Germany and elsewhere in 2011 were traced to a single lot of infected fenugreek seeds originating in Egypt. Exposure to even a small quantity of the seeds/sprouts can have a severe health impact and mortality is not insignificant (European Food Safety Authority).

5. B. *S. typhi* is unique among *Salmonella* spp. in having humans as its only reservoir. Boiling immediately destroys *S. typhi* by denaturing its thermolabile V antigen.

6. A. As might be expected diarrhoea is by far the most common problem reported and is also the most common problem for the ordinary tourist.

7. C. Campylobacter resistance to FQs is rapidly increasing not only in Thailand but also in other Asian countries. Azithromycin either Ig for 1 day or 500 mg daily for 3 days can be successful in treating the Campylobacter infection.

8. B. The rising rates of Campylobacter diarrhoea were recognized as far back as 2003 in Nepal when the primary enteric pathogens for tourists were Campylobacter (20%), Shigella (20%), ETEC (14%), Rotavirus (13%), Giardia (11%), Aeromonas (10%), and Cyclospora and related (5%). One study reports that up to 85% of diarrhoea in Thailand is now due to Campylobacter.

9. B. Campylobacter is sensitive to stomach HCl. Achlorhydria from any cause can reduce the minimum infective dose to well below the usual 10,000 organisms. Most human infections result from the consumption of improperly cooked, or poorly cleaned or contaminated foodstuffs. Chickens probably account for 50–70% of infections.

Other routes of transmission are faeco-oral, person-to-person, sexual contact, raw milk, contaminated water supplies, and close association with sick pets, especially puppies.

Bacteraemia can occur particularly in those with HIV/AIDS. In most colonized animals a lifelong carrier state develops.

10. B. Prolonged TD is most often due to a protozoal infection such as giardiasis or amoebiasis. Less often it is due to other protozoa such as cryptosporidia, cyclospora, or isospora. Far less frequently one of the other three options can cause prolonged TD.

11. C. Usually it takes over 108 CFUs to initiate clinical cholera unless the patient is debilitated, hypochlorhydric, or on proton pump inhibitors. Cholera toxin causes a secretory diarrhoea with little or no mucosal inflammation. Biotype 0139 was discovered in 1992 in Chennai. So far it is primarily confined to India and Bangladesh, and is only found in a minority of strains isolated elsewhere, e.g. in Thailand. Biotype 0139 emerges seasonally in an erratic manner without yet causing a feared pandemic. About 95% of diarrhoea due to cholera is mild and indistinguishable from other causes of TD.

12. A. Both cholera and ETEC attach to the villi of the small intestine but only ETEC penetrates as far as the submucosa.

The cholera toxin is the prototype of enterotoxins. It consists of a central A molecule (the toxin) surrounded by five molecules (like five fingers) which constitute the B subunit. It is the B subunit that attaches to the gut mucosa and presents the toxic core (the A moiety) to the cell. Here the A toxin stimulates cAMP so that chloride channels are opened, thus causing the outpouring of NaCl and water into the lumen of the gut, namely a secretory diarrhoea.

The mechanisms by which E. coli causes human diarrhoea are by synthesis of shigella dysenteriae-like enterotoxins, by invasion of the intestinal mucosa, and by unknown pathways. The B subunit of cholera bears an astonishing resemblance to the ETEC enterotoxin. The genesis of vomiting in TD is unknown.

13. A. C. difficile is a major cause of pseudomembranous colitis and antibiotic-associated diarrhoea. It thrives when there is an interference with the normal intestinal flora and causes frequent foul-smelling watery stools. Avoid unnecessary or prolonged antibiotics and use Imodium™ and Lomotil™ judiciously. Probiotics can be helpful in C. difficile enteritis as they tend to restore normal gastrointestinal flora (see below).

14. D. C. difficile is a motile anaerobic bacterium which, when stressed, forms spores. It can live in vitro for 70 days and can be carried from one person to another by hands or fomites. C. difficile is a commensal organism of the gut, present in 2–5% of healthy adults. However, it can account for up to 50% of the normal gut flora in under 2-year-olds. Personal hygiene and scrubbing of surfaces with bleach prevents its spread. *C. difficile* can flourish not only after antibiotic treatment, but also after repeated enemas, prolonged nasogastric tube usage, or gastrointestinal surgery.

15. B. *G. lamblia* is the most likely organism to cause these symptoms, but they can occur with any of the others listed above, which often exist as co-pathogens.

Note there is still doubt whether *Blastocystis hominis* (common in the stool of visitors to developing countries) is pathogenic to humans.

16. A. Humans are the main reservoir for giardia. The contribution made by cats and dogs is not known. Good hygiene and sanitation would almost certainly eliminate the human disease.

17. C. *Aeromonas* spp. causes about 2% of TD in travellers to Africa, Asia, and Latin America. It typically causes watery non-bloody diarrhoea that can persist for over a year. Spanish workers reported that 50% of those affected also suffered from fever and abdominal cramps. They found that cefotaxime (third generation cephalosporin), ciprofloxacin, and nalidixic acid were the best agents for treating the condition. Ampicillin was ineffective. *E. coli* is the most common cause of TD in Mexico (CDC 2011).

18. D. *D. fragilis* is a single-cell non-flagellate trichomonad parasite found in the colon and rectum of humans, pigs, and gorillas. It has worldwide distribution. It is unusual in that it has no cyst stage. Infective trophozoites survive only a short time when excreted in the faeces, hence the word 'fragilis'. Infection is generally faeco-oral and most likely acquired by eating in places manned by unhygienic staff. Only a small number of affected adults manifest the disease (diarrhoea) whereas symptoms appear in 90% of colonized children. A study in Australian travellers in 2007 indicates that 10% of patients infected with *D. fragilis* acquired the infection while overseas so that this infestation should be borne in mind in all cases of persistent TD in travellers.

Recommended treatment for symptomatic patients includes tetracycline, metronidazole, carbarsone, iodoquinol, diphetarsone, erythromycin, hydroxychinoline, paromomycin, and secnidazole. Chronic infections also occur and may present with intermittent diarrhoea, vague abdominal pain, and weight loss.

19. D. One survey in 28 developing countries, using Spain as a base line with a reporting rate ratio (RRR) of 1.0, showed the risk of TD was highest in Nepal with an RRR of 669.9. Other RRRs were India 542.3, Peru 227.5, Kenya 203.2, Cuba 88.4, Philippines 71.7, Thailand 54.9, South Africa 23.4, Tunisia 22.6, Mexico 19.3, Turkey 9.2, and China 4.0.

20. A. The risk of Campylobacter or Salmonella is small in good tourist restaurants in Thailand. However, *Ar. butzleri* is very common in Bangkok with an exposure rate as high as 13% when eating in good restaurants and a likely 75% chance of acquiring it if >10 meals are eaten.

Arcobacter differs from Campylobacter in its ability to grow at lower temperatures and in air. Of the six *Arcobacter* spp. described, only *Ar. butzleri* is associated with human enteritis. While untreated water is a source of infection it is chiefly spread by contaminated food, especially poultry.

Arcobacter diarrhoea can be severe, blood stained, and prolonged. It responds to most antibiotics but is generally resistant to azithromycin, nalidixic acid, and trimethoprim-sulfamethoxazole. Note that Borrelia is not a cause of TD. *B. burgdorferi* is tick-borne and causes Lyme disease, and *B. recurrentis* is transmitted by human body lice and causes relapsing fever.

21. C. Rice as a substitute for glucose was first used successfully in India. Commercial rice-based preparations are now available, e.g. Ceralyte. ORS does not reduce stool frequency but replaces lost salt and water. Water is reabsorbed in the wake of sodium, which is itself co-transported with glucose via a shared symport on the luminal membrane of enterocytes. It is essential that ORS is never hypertonic to body fluids as this would draw water from gut to lumen. Normally each litre of ORS contains 3.5 g NaCl, 1.5 g KCl and 20 g glucose.

22. B. Enteropathogens carry antigens similar to human blood groups and this is the basis for the greater susceptibility of some people to certain microorganisms. The association of group A and giardiasis has an odds ratio of 0.2–0.8. The other options, as well as norovirus, appear to be more frequent in those with blood group O (odds ratios from 1.2 to 11.8). Norovirus is less frequent in those with blood group B.

23. D. As few as 10 cysts of *G. lamblia* can initiate diarrhoea in a healthy adult. Hypomotility states resulting from either antiperistaltic drugs, e.g. diphenyoxylate/atropine, loperamide, or opiates, or from disease, e.g. diabetes mellitus, promote TD. This is because proper motility is a major way of removing microorganisms, especially from the proximal small intestine.

Achlorhydric states, immunocompromise, and alterations in gut flora, e.g. antibiotic-induced, also promote TD. Ingested *E. coli* should exceed 100,000 organisms and *V. cholerae* exceed 100 million in order to cause diarrhoea.

Prevention of TD

1. D. Probiotics have been shown to be very effective in preventing TD (see below). Theoretically the best strategy is to avoid potentially contaminated food and drink. This should be allied to good personal hygiene. In practice most people do not follow this advice.

Compliance with bismuth preparations often fails (6–8 tablets/day) and unless there are exceptional circumstances prophylactic antibiotics are discouraged because they may be misused, may not be appropriate for the organisms encountered, may engender resistance, or may promote superinfection.

A clean-looking table often fronts a filthy kitchen.

2. D. Most studies find that there is no real decrease in the percentage of travellers who get TD despite strict adherence to WHO precautions. This may be due to the ubiquity of enteropathogens in areas of poor hygiene and sanitation, unhygienic storage and preparation of food, and/or lack of conscientious hand-washing and utensil washing by the traveller as well as by the provider.

3. C. Organisms remain viable on one's hands for at least 30 minutes. This allows ample time for autoinoculation (transfer to nasal mucosa, conjunctiva, or mouth).

Only about 8% of people use soap and only 2% wash their hands for longer than 10 seconds when using rest rooms.

Clean-looking hard surfaces, e.g. door handles, telephones, and table tops, are more likely to transfer pathogens to our hands than clean dry cotton towels. This may seem surprising, but most of us have been confronted with the spectacle of a waiter or waitress wiping a dirty rag across a café table in a process more akin to plating bacteria than cleaning.

Probiotics, prebiotics, and TD

1. C. According to the WHO, probiotics are 'live microorganisms which when administered in adequate amounts confer a health benefit on the host'. The probiotics *Lactobacilli* and *Saccharomyces boulardii* (a yeast) help maintain, enhance, and re-establish the normal gut flora and thus help prevent and treat TD. In particular, lactobacilli acidify the gut and produce a pH inimical to many pathogenic organisms. Probiotics are also used widely in the treatment of *C. difficile*-associated diarrhoea. Studies in healthy elderly patients suggest that probiotics may enhance immunity and so allow vaccines to be more effective.

2. C. It has been well documented that probiotics can be useful in both the prevention and treatment of bacterial, but not viral, TD, especially in children. However, there are also reports in which probiotics were shown to worsen diarrhoea. It is suggested that when probiotics are used in cases of severe diarrhoea the extra oxygen used by the probiotic bacteria reduces that available to the gut mucosa. Probiotics are widely available in supermarkets everywhere. Their effect on URIs is not proven.

3. B. Prebiotics are non-digestible oligosaccharides of which oligofructose and inulin are outstanding examples. They were named 'prebiotics' by Marcel Roberfroid in 1995. They increase the number/activity of healthy colonic bacteria, notably lactobacilli and bifidobacteria, that is, probiotics.

Good natural sources or prebiotocs include unrefined cereals, selected vegetables (artichokes, chicory roots, garlic, onions), and breast milk. Their postulated health effects vary and include stimulation of probiotics, immune enhancement, anti-colon cancer, anti-hypertension, bowel motility regulation, and many other beneficial actions.

It is suggested that a primary mechanism for the health benefits of prebiotics is their stimulation of short-chain fatty acid production. In general they are heat resistant and thus not destroyed by cooking food.

Skin infestations and infections

1. D. The Koebner phenomenon is very common and may be precipitated by a variety of minor traumata such as sunburn, scratching, the arms of spectacles, and chafing of garments. It occurs in CL and in other common skin conditions, e.g. psoriasis, pityriasis rosea, lichen dermatoses, vitiligo, and eczema. CL also produces seedlings by direct inoculation of infective material (amistogotes) to nearby sites in a fashion similar to the spread of warts and *Molluscum contagiosum* (viral particles). CL is transmitted by sandflies.

2. A. *L. braziliensis*, typically a cause of New World CL (NWCL) in South America, is not very susceptible to oral miltefosine, an agent that is useful in other types of CL. NWCL is far more likely to proceed to ML than OWCL. Unfortunately ML, also know as espundia, can be extremely disfiguring. Ninety per cent of all cases of ML occur in Bolivia, Brazil, and Peru. This mainly affects the nasal mucosa. Ten per cent of ML cases occur in the Old World, chiefly in southern Europe, the Middle East, and central Asia. These mainly affect the larynx and oral mucosa, and are due to *L. infantum*. OWCL also differs from the New World type in that it often heals spontaneously and seldom starts as CL.

The Leishmanin test, in which killed promastigotes are injected intradermally, is generally positive after 48 hours in CL and ML and is useful in travellers, provided the material used is area and type specific. The test is negative in VL.

Leishmaniasis recidivans is a chronic form of CL seen in Iraq and Iran, especially in children. Most cases are due to *L. tropica*. It persists intermittently for 20–40 years, usually on the face and often with scarring. Clinically it resembles lupus vulgaris (cutaneous TB).

Note the large increase in CL cases now appearing in travellers.

3. C. The CL lesion starts as a macule, progresses to a papule and nodule, and then ulcerates. If uninfected the lesion is typically painless. The Leishmanin test can be helpful if positive but it may also be positive in lupus vulgaris and a negative test may occur in the presence of early CL. An eosinophilia is not found unless there is a concomitant helminthiasis. Insect bites are so common in those travelling in endemic areas that such a history is rarely helpful.

4. A. Males and non-fertilized females feed intermittently on warm-blooded animals (domestic animals, rodents, wild animals) as well as on humans. Females penetrate the skin and burrow just as far as the dermis. Only the anus, copulatory organs, and four little air holes are exposed to the outside environment. Male fleas are attracted to and fertilize the embedded female. The males then die. Thousands of eggs mature while the female sustains itself by taking blood from local capillaries. These eggs are then discharged to the outside.

T. penetrans is endemic in tropical regions and thrives best on dry warm sandy soil, including beaches. It is believed that tungiasis is one of the few parasitic diseases that spread from the Americas eastward to Europe and Africa in the 19th century. *T. penetrans* is a strict ectoparasite.

5. D. Eggs hatch on the ground and pupate just under the sand or soil surface. They emerge from their larval cocoons as adults in 9–15 days. Adult fleas then seek a suitable host for food or in which to embed and reproduce. This cycle lasts 3–4 weeks.

The flea is a poor jumper and so is found mainly in the soft region between toes or under the nails but can affect any part of the body with which it is in contact. Multiple infestations are common. Children are at particular risk because they have less keratinization of the skin and are more likely to go barefoot. Treatment is by surgical excision of the flea and antibiotics for secondary infection. Ivermectin orally or topically (0.08% lotion) has also had good success. Tetanus toxoid may be indicated, especially in refugees. Tungiasis is extremely common in many tropical countries.

6. C. Myiasis is due to penetration of the intact skin by the larvae of a variety of two-winged flies (diptera). Human infestation is most commonly caused in Africa by the larvae of the tumbu fly (*Cordylobia anthrophaga*) and in Central and South America by the larvae of the human botfly (*Dermatobia hominis*) locally known as torcel, el torsalo, or ver macaque. The fly-deposited eggs develop into larvae on warm skin that they then penetrate and, if undisturbed, form furuncle-like lesions in which they further develop. Finally the lesions burst and fully formed larvae—now recognizable maggots—emerge to become adult flies once more. Of 33 cases of *D. hominis* imported into Japan, 18 originated in Brazil (2007).

7. D. Because the 'head' is the only way the larva gets oxygen then logical treatment consists of suffocating the larva by occluding it with oil or grease or with a strip of fatty bacon. After a few hours the larva emerges and is easy to remove. Careful removal is essential because of possible allergic reactions following larval break up during extraction. Anti-helminthic drugs are of no use.

African myiasis typically occurs on the trunk (eggs deposited on clothes) while the American variety occurs on the scalp and other exposed places (mosquito ferries eggs to humans). Myiasis can also present in unusual sites, e.g. penis, pharynx, rectum, and nose.

8. A. CLM is the most common tropical skin lesion found in travellers within a month of return from South-East Asia, Central and South America (including Mexico), or Africa. It is caused by penetration of the skin by a larva of *Ankylostoma braziliense* (hookworm) of dogs (*A. canis*), cats (*A. catis*), or other mammals. Usually this occurs when walking barefoot or sitting on beaches or on apparently clean hotel courtyards in hot countries. The larva may grow to 20 mm in length and advances a few millimetres per day. This contrasts with larva currens (*Strongyloides stercoralis*), where the rash is evanescent, often on the trunk rather than on legs or buttocks, and likely to appear years after exposure.

Gnathosyomiasis (larva migrans profundus) is a condition in which the larva of a *Gnathosoma* spp. (usually *G. spinigerum*) wanders around the body without completing its life cycle but lodges sometimes under the skin (intermittent painful migratory swellings), sometimes in other places (meninges, eye, muscle).

Humans are accidental hosts who generally acquire the parasite by ingesting third-stage larvae in undercooked or raw poultry, fish or frogs.

Calabar swelling (loa loa, the 'eye worm') is only acquired in West Africa. It is due to a local inflammatory/allergic reaction provoked by the presence of an adult worm migrating in the subcutaneous tissues. The reaction is greater if the worm is traumatized or partly disintegrates. The worm and its associated swelling progress at 0.5–1 cm/minute. Frequently the worm crosses the subconjunctival space, where it can be extracted surgically. This gives as much pleasure to the doctor as to the patient.

Moving subcutaneous skin lesions

1. Answers: A-9; B-10; C-10; D-8; E-5; F-6; G-7; H-5
   a. Ingestion of the larvae of dog/cat round worms causes toxocariasis.
   b. Migratory subcutaneous swellings characteristic of visceral gnathosyomiasis, larva currens profundus
   c. Subconjunctival passage of adult worms gives the name 'eye worm' to loiasis.
   d. Larva currens. Transient motile evanescent swellings. Neither onchocercal nodules nor the lesions of tungiasis move. These are the two odd men out.

Malaria

1. A. In one report it was found that none of 21 Americans who died from malaria had received an appropriate chemoprophylactic. In 62% of cases the physician missed the initial diagnosis while in 43% of cases the laboratory missed or misdiagnosed the condition. In over half the cases treatment was incorrect either as a drug choice or by the route of administration, e.g. oral quinine in severe malaria.

2. D. Latent liver forms (hypnozoites) of *P. vivax* and/or *P. ovale* can cause clinical attacks of malaria for months or years. *P. falciparum*, *P. malariae*, and *P. knowlesi* do not generate hypnozites. Recrudescence of infection caused by *P. falciparum* results from persisting blood forms in inadequately treated patients.

3. B. The usual ES for malaria is 6–28 days, although it can sometimes first present many years later especially, but not exclusively, if non-falciparum.

4. B. It has been shown in both Italy and France that a high level of antimalarial antibodies remains after 15 years in African immigrants who have not returned to malarial areas in the interim. Such 'semi-immune' subjects have a lower parasitemia, a quicker parasite clearance after treatment, and a significantly shorter fever time than non-immune subjects. Children of immigrants from an endemic area who are born in non-malaria countries have no immunity to malaria.

5. A. Although rare, splenic rupture is more common in vivax than in falciparum malaria. Nowadays splenic rupture is treated conservatively unless there is serious haemodynamic instability. Although a palpable asymptomatic spleen is present within 3–4 days of the onset of malaria in up to 90% of cases, a palpable spleen is not commonly found in cases of rupture (personal observation). Malaria is the most common tropical infectious agent that causes spontaneous splenic rupture.

6. A. The likelihood ratio for a positive diagnosis of malaria is 13.6 for splenomegaly, 11.0 for thrombocytopenia <150 mm³, and 4.6 for Hb <12.0 g/dl. Start anti-malaria treatment if no other diagnosis is established.

7. A. It makes sense that in such a potentially lethal condition one should have results to hand within 3 hours. Treatment should never be deferred longer than this if there is a high index of suspicion. Many physicians start malaria treatment as soon as blood has been taken from the patient and sent for examination.

Rapid diagnostic tests (RDTs)

1. A. RDT kits contain antibodies that react with parasite-specific histidine-rich protein-2 antigen (HRP-2) or with parasite-induced aldolase or with plasmodium lactate dehydrogenase (pLDH). HRP-2 is specific for *P. falciparum*, aldolase antibodies are pan-specific, detecting all types of malarial parasite but not differentiating between them. pLDH can be specific for either *P. falciparum* or *Plasmodiium vivax* or for any specific pathogenic plasmodium. There is no significant difference in the accuracy of any brand within these categories. Combi tests can be used to identify both *P. falciparum* and *P. vivax*.

Results are read within 15 minutes, but since a test can remain positive for up to 28 days after treatment, RDTs cannot be used to assess parasite clearance (Abba et al. 2011). RDTs should be backed up by direct microscopy of thin and thick films where possible. This is because of technical errors, out of date reagents, misinterpretation of the results, and false negatives when using RDTs.

2. D. Jelinek showed that 87% of tourists were unable to interpret the result correctly, 71% were unable to draw blood, 58% were unable to identify the bands, 39% did not wait the recommended time, and 26% were unable to place blood correctly on the kit. All these problems may be compounded if the kit is damaged. In particular pLDH-based kits are thermolabile. Note that Jelinek's study was based on only 33 travellers.

A study from the University of Zurich on Swiss subjects prior to travel showed that interpretation of RDTs (ParaSightF, MalaQ, ICT) was particularly poor when parasitaemia was <0.1%, that is, false negatives are liable to occur.

3. B. The greatest benefit of an RDT is the immediate diagnosis of serious *P. falciparum* malaria. However, false negative results can occur even at high parasitaemias, so that some argue it is better to assume malaria is present if someone in a malarious area shows signs and symptoms consistent with malaria, rather than rely on an RDT.

Recall that SBET should only be used when medical help is more than 24 hours away. Only targeted lay people should be trained to do the test. It is not indicated for the majority of travellers. Furthermore, when the index of suspicion is high, repeat tests should be performed. RDTs are useful in places where microscopy is absent or poor, as a diagnostic adjunct in centres that see returned travellers, and in doctors' surgeries where occassionally febrile returned travellers present themselves. In all cases RDTs should be done and read by trained personnel. Cost is seldom a deterrent except in very poor countries.

Retrospective diagnosis of malaria

1. B. The retrospective diagnosis of malaria is important for several reasons. Firstly there is the need to screen potential blood donors, secondly there is the need to ascertain if an individual is harbouring the hypnozoite stage of *P. ovale* or *P. vivax*, and thirdly there is the need to clarify whether or not a returned non-immune traveller, who has been treated for malaria in an endemic country, really had malaria. The IFAT test using blood-stage antigens is extremely sensitive in detecting malaria antibodies against *P. falciparum* and *P. vivax*. However, IFAT is not of use in diagnosing acute malaria and only becomes it positive 8–180 days after an attack.

A well-researched report from Munich on 105 travellers treated for malaria while in endemic areas showed that only 15% were IFAT positive for malarial antibodies. This indicates that malaria was originally misdiagnosed in 85% of these travellers while overseas, and is clearly a serious indictment of unnecessary and potentially dangerous treatment.

Filariasis

1. D. Lymphatic filariasis is transmitted by mosquitoes. It is caused by infection with two major nematode (round worm) parasites, *Wuchereria bancrofti* and *Brugia malayi*. *W. bancrofti* is transmitted from person to person by culex, aedes, and, especially in West Africa, anopheles mosquitoes. Mansonia mosquitoes are the main vectors for *B. malayi*. Both have almost identical life cycles in humans but *B. malayi* can also infect animals and has a reservoir in monkeys and cats whereas *W. bancrofti* has no zoonotic host. *W. bancrofti* is found throughout the tropics, *B. malayi* is confined to Asia. *Cx. quinquefasciatus*, the chief vector of *W. Bancrofti*, breeds mainly in drains, cess pits, and water that is polluted with rotting vegetation or sewage. It is therefore mainly an urban rather than a rural problem.

In contrast to anopheles and malaria both sexes of culex bite animals or humans for a blood feed, and both sexes deposit third-stage infective larvae on the skin during a blood feed. These enter the body through a nearby abrasion or the puncture wound made by the mosquito's proboscis. They then disseminate widely and finally lodge in lymph nodes where they mature after 6–12 weeks. Females release >100,000 sheathed microfilariae per day for up to 6 years.

Bites are timed to coincide with maximum amounts of microfilariae in the person's blood and this usually occurs at night time (nocturnal periodicity). *Brugian filariasis* (Asian filariasis) is generally less severe than the bancroftian variety that predominates in Africa. *Brugia timori* is confined to Indonesia. It causes a similar clinical picture to B. *malayi* and is treated in the same way. Both have a nocturnal perioidicity. *Onchocerca volvulus*, also a filaria, causes 'river blindness'. It is transmitted by the blackfly (*Simulium damnosum*), which usually breeds in fairly rapidly flowing water.

2. C. While LF may be asymptomatic in some expatriates and visitors it is more commonly associated with an acute onset of fever, painful lymph nodes (often in the groin), lymphangitis, and oedema of the bitten part, e.g. a limb. Genital involvement (testicular pain, hydrocoele, scrotal oedema) is also seen in bancroftian filariasis.

Microflariae only appear in the blood once the disease is well established. Current anti-LF drugs (diethycarbamazine citrate DEC, ivermectin, albendazole) are microfilaricidal and so reduce the prevalence of filarial disease in an endemic area. DEC and albendazole also damage the adult worm.

3. D. Eosinophilia occurs early in the disease but is so non-specific as to be of little help. The mosquito injects larvae into the victim but it is the microflariae produced by the adult worms that are subsequently found in the blood. Nocturnal periodicity is most common when the microfilariae become sequestered in the pulmonary capillaries by day. In parts of the Pacific and in some Polynesian islands microfilaremia is found during daylight to suit the biting habits of local mosquitoes (diurnal subperiodic). However, most symptomatic patients and non-symptomatic carriers do not have an observed microfilaraemia. ICT tests, based on monoclonal antibodies to filarial worms, are currently the most reliable way to make the diagnosis. The DEC provocative test is a diagnostic tool used to induce parasitaemia and thus exacerbate symptoms. It should be used with extreme caution in case it provokes an allergic hypersensitive reaction to the massive release of antigen from dying microfilariae (the Mazotti reaction). This can be life-threatening if the patient is coinfected with onchocerciasis. DEC kills both microfilariae and adults, and prior treatment with ivermectin 150 µg/kg reduces the danger of a Mazotti reaction.

Sexually transmitted infections (STIs)

1. C. Five per cent is an overall figure. The percentage is much higher in younger people, especially young males. Females are sexually active too, with up to 25% of young female inter-rail travellers from Northern Europe admitting to having had at least one casual sexual contact with an unknown partner while abroad. Alarmingly, one survey showed that >50% of men who have had sex with men overseas convert to HIV+ in under 2 years. The typical sex tourist is a male with a mean age of 38 years.

2. A. Vaginal candidiasis is very common in hot moist climates and is easily transmitted sexually. In females it causes a distressing itch and vaginal discharge, while in their male partners it causes an irritating balanitis. Hepatitis B is 100 times more transmissible than HIV and, like other

STIs, both are more easily transmitted sexually in the presence of genital ulceration, warts, inflammation, or mucosal erosions. Hepatitis C and D can also be transmitted sexually.

Other STIs facing the sexually active include gonorrhoea, papilloma viruses, *Trichomonas vaginalis*, herpes virus, *Haemophilus ducreyi* (chancroid), and lymphogranuloma venereum due to *Chlamydia trachomatis*.

'Travel' sex is often experimental and thus conjunctivitis and 'gay mans colitis' and all the common enteropathogens are seen on return. Syphilis (*Treponema pallidum*) is on the increase, particularly in Eastern Europe, and is being spread widely by migratory prostitutes.

Remember that anal sex, casual sex, and paid prostitution are rampant in many tourist destinations.

3. C. It is difficult to get an accurate figure. For example, in Nepal and in many Indian cities serology for syphilis in prostitutes is in the region of 20% while in the Baltic states it varies from 7% to 9%. Even in the USA there has been a steady rise in syphilis rates since 2000, with thousands of new cases being reported annually. The majority of these occurred in men who had sex with men. Patients should be warned of the very high risk of unprotected or experimental sex, especially when overseas.

4. A. It is impossible to be sure of the rate in many developing countries but it is very high in South-East Asian brothels and has been reported to be >80% in parts of Eastern Europe.

5. C. Any of these problems may face her but the risk of HIV is by far the most serious.

6. B. The overwhelming danger of HIV with doubtful sex in Uganda means that HAART is the preferred option (personal view). Other STIs are also common in such a situation, but it is unlikely that she is pregnant since intercourse occurred during menstruation and a condom, although of unknown quality, was allegedly used.

7. A. Any of these can act as opportunistic infections in immunocompromised people but *P. jirovecii* is the most common. Patients with CD4 counts less than 200 cells per mm^3 are most commonly affected. Prophylaxis with dapsone or the use of inhaled pentamidine and oral trimethoprim-sulfamethoxazole dramatically decrease the risk of this opportunistic infection.

Vaginal and/or oral thrush is probably the next most common infection. *T. gondii* infection can occur via ingestion of tissue cysts in undercooked game or raw meats and may result in weight loss and fever or manifest itself as a chorioretinitis, lymphadenitis, or even myocarditis. It is usually diagnosed by immunological tests and treated by sulfadiazine and pyrimethamine.

Motion sickness

1. C. Many studies confirm the usefulness of controlled breathing in preventing or ameliorating the symptoms of motion sickness. Sitting at the front of a car or bus or amidships in a boat or over the wings in an aeroplane is also helpful. Other recommendations include focusing on a distant object, closing one's eyes, and avoiding reading.

2. D. Men seem to be less likely to get motion sickness (mal-de-mer) than others. Children >2 years old, pregnancy, women near period time, and aerobically trained persons appear to be more at risk.

Dengue fever

1. **Which of the following is true of dengue virus (DV) and dengue fever?**
   A. DV has six major pathogenic serotypes
   B. Dengue fever is now endemic in most of southern Europe
   C. Serotype 3 (DENV-3) is spreading rapidly
   D. Dengue fever is very rare in travellers

2. **The usual maximum incubation period for dengue fever is**
   A. 2 weeks
   B. 2 months
   C. 12 months
   D. 24 months

3. **Dengue fever**
   A. Is more likely to occur in cities than in rural areas
   B. Is most likely acquired during the periods of dawn and dusk
   C. Is predominantly carried by the culex mosquito
   D. Is unusual in South America

4. **Which of the following is true of dengue fever?**
   A. A falling haematocrit ratio (HCT) is a serious sign in dengue fever
   B. A positive tourniquet test is a serious sign in dengue fever
   C. Dengue fever is more likely to be serious in poorly nourished than in well-nourished children
   D. Barrier nursing, if available, should always be used in cases of dengue fever

5. **Which of the following is also true of dengue fever?**
   A. Is less common than malaria in South-East Asia
   B. Is only manifest in humans
   C. Has been eliminated from major South American cities
   D. Is accompanied by a rash in over 75% of cases

6. **When doing the the tourniquet test**
   A. Ensure that the pressure is maintained at mean arterial pressure below the knee for 2 minutes and note the number of petechiae that appear below the level of compression
   B. Apply the tourniquet to either the upper arm or the upper leg
   C. Apply to a limb for 5 minutes and note the number of petechiae that appear below the level of compression
   D. Apply tourniquet as in C and count the number of petechiae per square inch below the level of compression

7. **An ominous signs in the course of dengue fever is**
   A. A sudden fall in fever
   B. A truncal rash
   C. A rise in C reactive protein (CRP)
   D. The onset of severe arthralgia

8. **Antibody-dependent enhancement (ADE)**
   A. Refers to protection from a second attack of dengue fever by the same DV serotype
   B. Refers to the brief heterologous cross-protection induced by a particular DV serotype
   C. Is a phenomenon shared by many viruses
   D. Helps protect humans against dengue

9. **Chikungunya fever**
   A. Is caused by a flavivirus
   B. Has a moderate mortality when acquired by non-immune adults, e.g. Western tourists
   C. Is co-located with dengue fever in many areas
   D. Is transmitted by both culex and anopheles mosquitoes

Enteric fever

1. **Enteric fever (syn. typhoid and paratyphoid fever)**
   A. Is largely prevented by Vi polysaccharide typhoid vaccine
   B. Responds well to trimethoprim/sulfamethoxazole (co-trimoxazole)
   C. Responds best to ciprofloxacin
   D. Is mostly caused by S. paratyphi in travellers

2. **Which of the following is true of enteric fever (serotype S. typhi and S. paratyphi)?**
   A. The critical infective dose of S. paratyphi is far less than that for S. typhi
   B. Sub-saharan Africa is the most common place to acquire S. paratyphi
   C. In typhoid endemic countries S. typhi infection is 10–20 times more common than paratyphoid infection
   D. Gender is an important risk factor for enteric fever

3. **The perpetuation of typhoid fever is ultimately due to**
    A. Infected faeces or urine of carriers or those currently ill from *S. typhi*
    B. Ingestion of seafood from infected waters
    C. The 'filthy feet of faecal-feeding flies'
    D. The persistence of *S. typhi* in water, ice, dust, and sewage

4. **The diagnosis of typhoid fever depends on**
    A. Culture of *S. typhi* from blood, urine, or stool
    B. A strongly positive Widal test
    C. Typical clinical signs
    D. The presence of clinical findings such as fever, headache, abdominal pain, and constipation in anyone who has recently returned from an endemic area

Miscellaneous

1. **Pathogenic brucella organisms survive in ice-cream for**
    A. 1 week
    B. 4 weeks
    C. 10 weeks
    D. 1 year

2. **Which of these is non-pathogenic?**
    A. *Entamoeba coli*
    B. Shigella dysenteriae
    C. *Campylobacter jejuni*
    D. ETEC

3. **Legionnaire's disease**
    A. Is caused by *Pneumocystis jirovecii* (*P. carinii*)
    B. Is highly contagious in the early stages of the disease
    C. Can be diagnosed by using a urinary antigen test
    D. Is susceptible to most antibiotics

4. **Which of the following is true on Legionnaire's disease?**
    A. Legionnaire's disease was first described in members of the French Foreign Legion serving in North Africa
    B. Legionnaire's disease is most likely to be contracted by ingestion of contaminated warm water, e.g. in spas or swimming pools
    C. Even if untreated, has a very small mortality except in special groups (infants, elderly, immunocompromised)
    D. The diagnosis is suggested by the failure of a pneumonia to respond to β-lactams or aminoglycosides

5. **The quickest way to diagnose brucellosis in a returned traveller with a pyrexia of unknown origin (PUO) is to**
   A. Grow the organism from blood culture
   B. Use a serum agglutination test (SAT)
   C. Perform a Coombs test
   D. Find involvement of the reticuloendothelial system (lymph nodes, liver, spleen)

6. **Which of the following is true of Salmonella?**
   A. Salmonella are mainly transmitted to humans via contaminated water
   B. Salmonella multiply rapidly in tropical sea water
   C. Salmonella are destroyed by modern sewage treating processes
   D. Salmonella are destroyed at temperatures in excess of 70°C

7. **Which of the following is true of Salmonella and human disease?**
   A. Most salmonella are pathogenic to humans
   B. Salmonellosis can cause Reiter's syndrome
   C. Contaminated foods usually look or smell abnormal ('off')
   D. Salmonella are so-called because they were first found in salmon

8. *Hemophilus influenzae*
   A. Has been found in the nasal secretions of up to 90% of healthy individuals worldwide
   B. Can cause eosinophilic meningitis in travellers
   C. Is also known as *Neisseria meningitidis*
   D. Is a virus

9. **Meningitis in travellers is mainly due to**
   A. *Haemophilus influenzae*
   B. *Neisseria meningitidis* (syn. meningococcus)
   C. Viral infections
   D. *Mycobacterium tuberculosis*

10. **Eosinophilic meningitis (EM) is typical of**
    A. Toscana virus infection
    B. *Angiostrongylus cantonensis* (rat lungworm)
    C. Aseptic meningitis
    D. Pulmonary eosinophilia (Loeffler's syndrome)

11. **Which of the following is true of *Giardia lamblia*?**
    A. *Giardia lamblia* is a multicellular protozoan
    B. *Giardia lamblia* has cysts that resist chlorination
    C. Large numbers of cysts must be ingested in order to cause infection
    D. *Giardia lamblia* chiefly affects the large intestine

12. **Which of the following is true of giardiasis?**
    A. Giardiasis has an incubation period of 3–6 weeks
    B. Giardiasis is sometimes associated with fleeting arthralgia
    C. Giardiasis may cause substantial weight loss and malabsorption
    D. Giardiasis lodges in the gall bladder in asymptomatic carriers

13. **The most important treatment for patients with moderate or severe cholera is**
    A. Administration of ORS
    B. IV fluid and electrolyte replacement
    C. Vigorous antibiotic therapy
    D. Full use of antidiarrhoeal medicines such as loperamide

14. **Cancer of the liver may be a long-term consequence of**
    A. Hepatitis A
    B. Amoebic liver disease
    C. Hydatid disease of the liver
    D. Oriental liver flukes

15. **Which of the following is true of schistosomiasis?**
    A. Schistosomiasis can be acquired by swimming in slow-flowing salt water
    B. Schistosomiasis can be acquired by swimming in the estuaries of some African rivers
    C. Schistosomiasis can be found in many chlorinated hotel pools
    D. Schistosomiasis is prevented if one wears a wet suit

16. **Lymphatic filariasis (LF) is transmitted by**
    A. Ticks
    B. Mosquitoes
    C. Swimming in stagnant water
    D. Inhalation

17. **Koplik spots occur in**
    A. Acute HIV pharyngitis
    B. Melioidosis
    C. Measles
    D. Diphtheria

18. **Which of the following conditions is transmitted to humans by rubbing infected vector faeces into the skin puncture?**
    A. Malaria
    B. Leishmaniasis
    C. Chagas' disease (American trypanosomiasis)
    D. Yellow fever

19. **West Nile virus (WNV)**
   A. Is generally confined to areas of Africa west of the river Nile
   B. Is normally transmitted by a tick bite
   C. Is sometimes transmitted sexually
   D. Is believed to have been introduced to America from Israel

20. **WNV can be transmitted to humans from**
   A. Direct contact with birds
   B. Direct contact with fowl
   C. Blood transfusion
   D. Close contact with patients who have active WNV

21. **WNV is most commonly carried by**
   A. Bats
   B. Crows and jays
   C. Spiders
   D. Dogs and cats

22. **Death most often occurs in West Nile encephalitis in**
   A. The elderly
   B. Children
   C. Women of child-bearing age
   D. Rural rather than city dwellers

23. **Gnathosyomiasis is most likely to occur in**
   A. Thailand
   B. Brazil
   C. Northern Australia
   D. India

24. **Eating raw or partly cooked fish in Thailand is associated with**
   A. Gnathosyomiasis
   B. Schistosomiasis
   C. Filariasis
   D. Ascariasis

25. *Taenia saginata* **(beef tapeworm)**
   A. Is more evenly distributed worldwide than *T. solium*
   B. Uses humans as its definitive host
   C. May cause neurocysticercosis
   D. May occur after eating unwashed vegetables

26. Which of the following are transmitted by ticks?

A. Hantavirus
B. Ehrlichiosis
C. Toxocariasis
D. Melioidosis

27. Melioidosis is chiefly acquired

A. Percutaneously from exposure to contaminated soil or mud
B. By ingesting unpasteurized dairy products
C. By living in rat-infested areas
D. By handling infected fowl, e.g. chickens, ducks

28. Which of the following is true of melioidosis?

A. Melioidosis may mimic pulmonary TB
B. Melioidosis is readily cured using a tetracycline, e.g. doxycycline
C. Most serologically positive persons are symptomatic
D. Melioidosis is a rare cause of pneumonia in Thailand

29. Which of the following is transmitted by sandflies?

A. Oroya fever (Carrion's disease)
B. Thalassaemia
C. Q fever
D. Plague

30. What is the principal reservoir for *Coxiella burnetti* (Q fever)?

A. Wild deer
B. Rodents
C. Domestic and farm animals
D. Symptomless humans

31. Which of the following is true of Q fever?

A. Treat initially with quinolones or azithromycin
B. There is a vaccine available
C. Most patients develop intense itch
D. Q fever is mostly found in hot sandy places

32. Which of the following is a bacterium?

A. *Cryptosporidium parvum*
B. *Isospora belli*
C. *Cyclospora cayenatensis*
D. *Burkholderia pseudomallei*

33. Match the following symptoms/signs with the appropriate disease. Options may be used once, more than once, or not at all

A. Itching
B. Track-like subcutaneous lesions
C. Urticaria
D. Skin nodules
E. Papules
F. Furuncle-like lesion(s)

1. Dog hookworm
2. Myiasis
3. Onchocerciasis
4. Tungiasis
5. Leishmaniasis
6. Scabies

34. Kala-azar (VL) in India

A. Is confined to southern India
B. Is a strict zoonotic disease
C. Can be carried by ticks
D. Is frequently associated with post Kala-azar dermal leishmaniasis (PKDL)

35. Post Kala-azar dermal leishmaniasis

A. Only occurs in chronic cases of kala-azar
B. Is caused by a reaction to dead leishmania
C. Is associated with an enormous number of live leishmanial parasites in the skin
D. Is associated with multiple ulcerative skin lesions

36. Which of the following is true of leprosy?

A. BCG vaccination can confer some protection against leprosy
B. Reflexes are usually altered in lepromatous neuropathy
C. Leprosy has never been reported in anyone who has spent only a short time in an endemic area
D. Thalidomide is now a first-line drug in treating leprosy

37. Cutaneous diphtheria

A. Is prevented by prior vaccination against diphtheria
B. Usually progresses to systemic diphtheria
C. Is a complication of respiratory diphtheria
D. Is occasionally imported from developing countries

38. Tick paralysis is caused by

A. A virus carried by the tick
B. A bacteria carried by the tick
C. A toxin produced by the tick
D. An allergic reaction to the tick bite

39. A typical feature of a tick paralysis is

A. Ascending paralysis
B. Descending paralysis
C. Prodromal vomiting
D. Sparing of the respiratory muscles

40. Tick-borne encephalitis virus

A. Is an alpha virus
B. Has a declining habitat worldwide
C. Is also transmitted to humans by fleas
D. Is transmitted to humans within minutes of being bitten

41. Tick-borne encephalitis virus

A. Is readily destroyed by acidic human stomach contents
B. Is primarily dependent on ticks feeding on viraemic large animals (cattle, goats, sheep, dogs, cats)
C. Only lives in humans as an incidental host
D. Carries a similar mortality wherever it is contracted

42. The risk of developing Japanese encephalitis is greater in

A. Urban rather than rural areas
B. The monsoon season
C. Mountainous areas rather than the lowlands
D. South America than South-East Asia

43. Which of the following areas are known to be free from Japanese encephalitis?

A. Bali
B. Nepal
C. Australia
D. Western Russia

44. Which of the following is true of babesiosis?

A. Babesiosis occurs worldwide but especially in the tropics
B. Babesiosis is a fungal infection
C. Babesiosis is a special risk for cave explorers, bat observers, and miners
D. Babesiosis is transmitted to humans by *Ixodes* spp. (ticks)

Dengue fever

1. C. Dengue has four major serotypes, 1–4. DENV-3 subtype 111 is spreading rapidly, especially in South America, and seems to be the type most often associated with dengue haemorrhagic fever (DHF). However, during the Pakistan outbreak of 1994 DENV-2 was responsible for six of the seven DHF cases. The current dengue epidemic is spreading throughout the tropics and the vectors *Ae. aegypti* and *Ae. albopictus* are expanding their territories.

The failure of dengue fever to make a major impact in developed tropical countries is due to good housing, good mosquito control, and a low viraemia in the human population. It appears that indigenous black Africans have a genetic resistance to dengue fever, but it is becoming increasingly common in travellers.

2. A. It is important to know the ES of major diseases in the returned traveller. The ES of dengue fever is a maximum of 2 weeks. More commonly the ES is 3–5 days.

3. A. Dengue fever (breakbone fever) is predominantly a daytime urban disease transmitted by *Ae. aegypti* and *Ae. albopictus*. It is on the increase worldwide and is a spreading problem in South America. There are >250 million cases worldwide and at least 21,000 deaths.

4. B. Dengue fever is a VHF, thus increased capillary permeability with capillary leak is a feature. Progression to DHF is suspected if there is a positive tourniquet test, a rise in the HCT ratio, a progressive fall in the platelet count, and a sudden fall in temperature. It is proposed that well-nourished children who mount a very strong immunological response are more liable to serious clinical symptoms than those less able to mount a strong immunological response. Barrier nursing is not needed since dengue fever is not contagious.

The major VHFs are yellow fever, dengue fever, Crimean–Congo fever, Rift Valley fever, and Lassa, Ebola, Marburg, and Hantaan fevers.

5. B. Dengue fever is a unique VHF in that humans are the primary host. Dengue fever is at least three times more common than malaria in travellers returning from South-East Asia. Large confirmed outbreaks have been reported from South America, including in cities, e.g. Lima. A rash appears in less than 50% of cases and was absent in all cases in the Lima outbreak of 2010–11.

6. D. If the number of petechiae exceeds 20 per square inch then the test is positive. This is a most useful test of capillary integrity in dengue fever.

7. A. A sudden fall in fever, especially when coinciding with a rise in the HCT, is a sign of impending DHF. It reflects serious plasma leakage and interference with the thermoregulatory centres. CRP is elevated in most inflammatory processes and arthralgia is a fairly typical symptom of classical dengue fever. A rash occurs in <50% of cases.

8. C. A first attack of dengue fever confers immunity for some months against all four serovars of dengue. After that, life-long immunity is retained only against the initial serovar and exposure to any of the others is more likely to result in DHF than expected. ADE in dengue is said to occur when a second attack of DV by a different serotype facilitates infectivity of the new strain and increases the danger of DHF. The different strain does this by provoking abundant anti-viral antibodies against the original strain of DV which cross-react with but do not cross-neutralize the new strain of virus. The cross-reacting antibody coats the new strain of DV and allows it to enter macrophages where division of the virus proceeds apace.

Many viruses exhibit the ADE phenomenon, e.g. Ebola virus (especially the Zaire strain). Nonetheless the ADE theory is contested nowadays by many research workers. ADE was formerly known as immune enhancement. Dengue serovars appear and disappear from different areas in an erratic manner.

9. C. Chikungunya fever is only found in areas where dengue fever is endemic, although it is not present in every dengue endemic area. Both are carried by *Ae. aegypti* and *Ae. albopictus*. The condition was first described in Tanzania in 1955 but the virus, an alpha virus, was only isolated in 1958 in Thailand. Recently large outbreaks have occurred in India and in islands in the Indian Ocean (Mauritius, Seychelles, Réunion). These have caused considerable morbidity and contributed to mortality in older or debilitated subjects. Many cases occur in travellers.

There is sudden severe headache, severe flu-like symptoms, and typically an excruciating backache. Chikungunya fever and dengue fever are the most common arboviral infections to cause a rash. Symptoms of varying degrees of severity may last for over a year.

Enteric fever

1. D. Enteric fever is a worldwide disease caused by *Salmonella enterica* (*S. typhi* and *S. paratyphi* A, B and C) Nowadays *S. paratyphi* A has overtaken *S. typhi* as the chief cause.

Ceftriaxone (third-generation cephalosporin) is considered the drug of first choice in treating enteric fever. Resistance to nalidixic acid is a good marker for the rapidly emerging resistance to ciprofloxacin. It is a misconception that 'paratyphoid fever' due to *S. paratyphoid* A is always a milder disease than classical typhoid fever caused by *S. typhi*. Paratyphoid B is more common than paratyphoid A in Mediterranean areas, with the reverse being the case in Asia.

There is evidence that Ty21a live oral typhoid vaccine confers about 50% protection against paratyphoid B.

2. C. While typhoid is 10–20 times more common in those living in endemic areas the reverse is probably true for travellers. This is because close intimacy within households facilitates the easy spread of *S. typhi* to residents whereas travellers, except those VFRs, are more likely to be exposed to *S. paratyphi*-contaminated food from street vendors.The infective dose of typhoid is low (100 bacteria) compared to paratyphoid (about 1000 bacteria) but the latter can divide rapidly, thus contaminated food is a major vehicle for paratyphoid transmission. Enteric fevers are most commonly found in the Indian sub-continent. Gender is not a risk factor for enteric fever.

3. A. All the options listed are involved in the spread of S. typhi. However, infected human excretions are the ultimate cause of S. typhi persisting in the world. This is compounded by inadequate sewage disposal in many countries. The most common immediate source is probably poor personal hygiene with direct contamination of food or drink by the hands of carriers. S. typhi multiplies in seafood that thrives in polluted water.

4. A. A positive blood culture, or, more likely, a positive bone marrow culture in the first week of the illness is a sure way of making the diagnosis. In the second week positive stool or urine cultures may be expected. The Widal test is probably underused nowadays because is non-specific and is not very sensitive. There is no such thing as a typical history in typhoid fever. As often as not it presents as a PUO. The 'rose spot' rash is found in less than 50% of cases and diarrhoea is present more often than constipation. The differential diagnosis includes malaria, brucellosis, meningitis, amoebiasis, and typhus. The incubation period of typhoid is 7–21 days.

Miscellaneous

1. B. Do not eat ice-cream of doubtful origin.

2. A. Entamoeba coli is a non-pathogenic commensal protozoan. Some selected minimum infective doses in pathogenic organisms: Shigella 10, Campylobacter jejuni 500, most vibrios 10^4, ETEC 10^7 (not known for strain O157) Salmonella 10^5–10^7, Cryptosporidium parvum 10 cysts, E. histolytica 1–10 cysts, Listeria unknown.

3. C. L. pneumophila serogroup 1 is the < cause of Legionnaire's disease and is detected by a urinary antigen test which is fast, inexpensive, and approaches 70% sensitivity and 100% specificity. Unfortunately it does not detect other types, e.g. serogroup 6, which is frequent in children. There is no person-to-person transmission. Since L. pneumophila is an intracellular organism it is only susceptible to antibiotics that reach inhibitory concentrations in cells, e.g. quinolones, macrolides, ketolides, tetracyclines, and rifampin. Azithromycin is the antibiotic of choice in children, quinolones in adults. P. jirovecii (formerly P. carinii) is a fungus and an extracellular pathogen. It causes pneumonia in immunocompromised hosts.

4. D. Untreated, Legionnaire's disease can have a mortality rate of >30% and only antibiotics that reach high intracellular concentrations are effective, e.g. quinolones and azithromycin. Legionnaire's disease is transmitted by aerosolization or aspiration of water contaminated with legionella organisms. The organism will not grow outside the range of 20–60°C, although rarely cold water and even ice has been contaminated. In European hotels colonization of hot water systems by legionella varies between 25% and 75%. However, not all serogroups are harmful to humans.

5. B. SAT is rapid, sensitive (95.6%), and specific (100%) for bacteraemic brucellosis. A titre of 1/160 in a symptomatic patient in a non-endemic area is considered positive. The Coombs' test for blocking antibodies is useful but not diagnostic if the SAT is negative. Blood culture is the only definitive way of diagnosing brucellosis and is around 90% positive in the early but not late stages. B. melitensis accounts for about 90% of human infections in most parts of the world.

6. D. Some Salmonella spp. can survive heating to 50°C but all are destroyed >70°C. Infected food of animal origin (poultry, pigs, cattle) or dairy products (mayonnaise, cheese) and contaminated vegetables are the main sources of *Salmonella* spp. *Salmonella* spp. abound in sludge and slurry from humans and animals but are also found in treated sewage and are carried by fish, amphibians, molluscs, and crustaceans. Salmonella survive drying, salting, and freezing, and have a remarkable ability to thrive in fruit juice and withstand the acid of the human stomach.

7. B. Most of the known 2500 Salmonella species are non-pathogenic. Exceptions include *S. typhi*, *S. paratyphi*, *S. enteritidis*, and *S. typhimurium*, which can be important causes of diarrhoea, especially in the traveller. In addition they are becoming more and more resistant to antibiotics. In a minority of people chronic salmonellosis can cause Reiter's syndrome (arthritis, iritis, urethritis). This occurs irrespective of whether or not antibiotics are used. Contaminated food looks and tastes normal. Salmonella are called after the American scientist Daniel Salmon who discovered them in 1883.

8. A. *H. influenzae* is an extremely common commensal of the upper respiratory tract. It is a non-motile Gram-negative diplococcus identified in 1892 by Richard Pfeiffer during an influenza pandemic. It was then called Pfeiffer's bacillus. In 1933 the cause of influenza was recognized to be a virus not a bacterium.

H. influenzae type B (HiB) was the most common form of bacterial meningitis until effective vacciniation was introduced (1985). HiB along with Neisseria (meningococci) and streptococci account for >80% of bacterial meningitis.

9. B. On average 10% of populations in countries with endemic disease carry *Neisseria meningitidis* asymptomatically in the nose and throat. This rises to 25% in adolescents.

Meningococcal serogroups A, B, C, Y, and W-135 are based on the composition of the capsular polysaccharide. While B and C have been responsible for most disease in the Americas and Europe, serogroup A and, to a lesser extent, serogroup C account for most meningococcal disease in Africa and in some areas of Asia. Nowadays serogroup Y has emerged as a cause of disease in North America. The W-135 strain has been isolated in epidemics in Saudi Arabia and Burkina Faso, and currently rivals serogroup A in frequency in parts of Africa. There is no vaccine effective against type B meningogcoccus. Options A, C and D can also cause meningitis.

10. B. Eosinophilic meningitis is defined by the presence of 10 or more eosinophils per microlitre in the CSF or an eosinophilia of at least 10% of the total CSF leukocyte count. *Angiostrongylus cantonensis* (rat lungworm) is the most common cause, followed by gnathosyomiasis and coccidioidomycosis. Malignancies (Hodgkin's disease, non-Hodgkin's lymphoma, eosinophilic leukemia), medications (ciprofloxacin, ibuprofen, gentamicin), systemic disease (sarcoidosis), and allergies (radio-contrast dyes, intracerebral shunt, prostheses) are also to blame. Sometimes no cause is found. There are several reports of eosinophilic meningitis in travellers due to rat lungworm acquired by eating snails, frogs, prawns or vegetables infested with live larvae. Examples abound: French police returning from Polynesia; 12 of 23 tourists returning from Jamaica; a Belgian woman returned from Latin America and Fiji. Toscana viral infection is transmitted by sandflies and is especially prevalent in southern France and in Tuscany, Italy. Toscana neuroencephalitis is on the increase. Cerebral gnathosyomiasis is usually more severe, with a bloody CSF and marked CNS symptoms. Aseptic meninigitis is caused by non-bacterial organisms, e.g. viruses, fungi, spirochetes, and parasites.

11. B. Giardia lamblia is a single-celled protozoan that can survive for 2 months in cold water and can resist chlorination. When cysts reach the small intestine they develop into trophozites, some of which remain free while others attach firmly to the mucosa. Ingesting fewer than 10 cysts can cause infection. Giardiasis is a worldwide problem. It was first described in St Petersburg at the end of the 19th century.

12. C. Chronic cases are associated with villus atrophy in the small intestine and can cause serious weight loss and malabsorption. The incubation period is 3 days to 3 weeks. Asymptomatic carriers are common but the gallbladder is unaffected.

13. B. Immediate massive IV fluid replacement is mandatory. Death from fluid and electrolyte loss (hypovolaemic shock) can occur in under 2 hours in severe or what was initially labelled 'moderate' cholera. Drugs such as loperamide (Imodium™) and diphenoxylate (Lomotil™) have no place in these cases. The WHO recommends ORS for mild cases. Antibiotics can kill the vibrio and lessen the risk of further spread.

14. D. Oriental liver flukes, *Opisthorchis sinensis* (previously called *Clonorchis sinensis*) and *O. viverrini*, have a human and animal reservoir in Japan, South-East Asia and southern ex-USSR countries. The adults (hermaphrodites) live in the bile ducts of humans, from where eggs are passed into the faeces. Untreated faeces contaminate water. *O. sinensis* accounts for 15% of liver cancer in Hong Kong. The other choices are not applicable.

15. B. All four major types of schistosomiasis (*S. hematobium*, *S. mansoni*, *S. japonicum*, *S. intercalatum*) are acquired when free-living motile cercariae, which infest fresh water lakes, rivers, and estuaries, penetrate the skin. Wet suits do not offer protection. Schistosomiasis cannot survive in seawater or in properly chlorinated pools. Beware of doubtful hotel pools in endemic areas. Note that, unlike *S. hematobium* or *S. mansoni*, *S. intercalatum* is not associated with late-onset cancer in either bladder or colon.

16. B. Mosquitoes transmit LF. *W. bancrofti* is distributed widely in the tropics and accounts for about 90% of cases. *Brugia malayi* and *Brugia timori* are confined to India, eastern Asia, and the Pacific regions.

17. C. Koplik spots are distinct white areas easily seen on the buccal mucus membrane opposite the molar teeth in measles. They consist of necrotic areas infiltrated with mononuclear cells. Measles is extremely common in children who have not been vaccinated and is a highly lethal disease in malnourished children. The low uptake of measles vaccine in developed countries in recent times is of special concern for travellers to developing nations.

18. C. The reduviid, triatomine 'assassin', or 'kissing' bug must get a blood meal to fully mature. Both sexes bite at night, especially around the face, and this is usually a painless unnoticed episode. During its feed it passes faeces loaded with trypanosomes, e.g. *T. cruzi*,on to the skin or mucus membranes. One then unknowingly rubs this into the puncture wound or nearby abrasion. Louse borne typhus (*R. proazeki*) is also rubbed into a breach in the skin in a similar fashion.

19. D. WNV, a flavivirus, is widely distributed in Africa, Asia, the Middle East, and southern Europe. It first appeared as a cause of disease in New York in August 1999, where there were 62 confirmed cases and seven deaths. It spread rapidly to 40 states, Washington DC, and even to Canada, the Caribbean, and Mexico. Clusters in the region of JFK airport suggest that it was imported probably from Israel. Mosquitoes (*Culex pipiens*) carry the infection from infected birds and transmit the virus to humans and other animals when they bite. WNV causes fever, arthralgia, rash, and encephalitis. Serious illness carries a mortality of about 1/250, but 80% of those infected are asymptomatic.

WNV was first isolated from a febrile woman in Uganda in 1937. It was characterized in Egypt in the 1950s and recognized as a cause of severe meningoencephalitis in Israel in 1957.

20. C. Apart from bites from carrier culcicine mosquitoes and perhaps bites from 'bridge vectors' such as aedes, WNV can be transmitted by blood transfusion, platelet or red cell transfusion, organ transplant, and across the placenta. Since 2003 Canada has screened blood for WNV nucleic acid. In the USA alone there may be may be >400,000 silent seropositive people.

21. B. WNV is carried by over 200 species of birds, especially crows and jays. It is also found in dogs, cats, horses, cattle, rabbits, skunks, racoons, and many other vertebrates. The basic life cycle is mosquito–bird–mosquito. Human are an irregular dead-end host.

22. A. Death is due to neuroinvasive disease and the elderly are most at risk. The young recover much more quickly. In one New York outbreak most cases occurred in those >50 years of age and these had a death rate of 10–20%. However, the overall death rate is <4%. Multiple mosquito bites enhance the risk and urban dwellers who sleep or rest outdoors on hot summer evenings are easy prey.

23. A. Gnathosyomiasis is a helminth infection highly endemic in Thailand and in some parts of Japan. It is also found in other South-East Asian countries and in Latin America.

24. A. The larvae of *G. spinigerum* mature into encysted adults that live in the stomach wall of their definitive hosts, e.g. cats, dogs, tigers, leopards, frogs, poultry, and herons. The water flea (Cyclops) ingests ova which have been passed in faeces deposited near ponds and streams. The ova develop in the water flea, which is eaten by a fresh-water fish. Consequently there are many larval-infected fish ready for the market The precise life cycle in humans is unclear. Larvae wander throughout the body being manifest as discrete migratory subcutaneous swellings, 'larva migrans'. Lodgment and maturation in deeper organs also occurs. Indeed many cases of subconjunctival invasion have been reported where whole live adult worms have been extracted. Eosinophilia is frequent but not invariable. Drugs, e.g. albendazole or ivermectin, have little effect. A worrying spread to Central America and Mexico has occurred in recent years. Rarely *G. nipponicum*, *G. doloresi*, and *G. hispidium* (in pork) have also been shown to cause human disease. Humans are an unfortunate accidental dead-end host for gnathosyomiasis.

Ocular involvement is a feature of many worms' life cycles, especially nematodes. These include loa loa, dirofilia, mansonella, dracunculus, angiostrongylus, and *W. bancrofti*. Gnathosoma directly invade eye structures.

25. B. *T. saginata* (beef tapeworm) is worldwide whereas *T. solium* (pork tapeworm) only occurs in pork-eating countries. *T. saginata* is particularly common in Ethiopia, Kenya, and India. Humans are the definitive hosts and ultimately the only reservoir of infection. *T. solium* causes human cysticercosis. Neurocysticercosis is a common cause of epilepsy in Central America and India (see chapters 4 and 16). A single dose of PZQ (10–40 mg/kg) is the drug of choice for almost all intestinal cestode infestations.

26. B. Ehrlichiosis (a rickettsia) is transmitted by ticks. It may coexist in the same tick with the spirochete *Borrelia burgdoferi* (Lyme disease) and the flavivirus that causes tick-borne encephalitis. Ehrlichiosis was first described in 1990 and is now chiefly reported from the USA and Europe. It has also been reported in travellers to Mali and Thailand. It causes a flu-like illness but in severe cases renal failure and coagulopathies can occur. Like other rickettsial diseases it is treated with doxycycline.

Hantavirus is inhaled by humans from the aerosolized excreta of infected rats. It can have a high mortality, with lung and kidney damage prominent. *Toxocara catis* and *cani* are worldwide helminths causing disease mainly in children 2–7 years old. Up to 95% of healthy adults living in the tropics carry it. Transmission is by ingestion of anything contaminated by the toxocara ova that are found in the faeces of cats and dogs. Those who play with dogs and cats are most at risk. Infected sandpits are notorious sources of toxocara eggs.

27. A. Melioidosis (Whitmore's disease) is caused by *Burkholderia pseudomallei*, formerly called *Pseudomonas pseudomallei*. *B. pseudomallei* is a free-living aerobic Gram-negative motile flagellated saprophytic bacillus that thrives in mud, moist soil, and surface water in parts of South-East Asia, Australia, New Zealand, and Madagascar. Humans contract melioidosis by ingestion or from contaminated injuries or sometimes through unbroken skin. Acquisition via inhalation (rare) appears to carry the threat of serious disease. Clinically it ranges from being asymptomatic to an overwhelming septicaemia. Localized cutaneous and visceral abscesses with necrotizing pneumonia, osteomyelitis, and sepsis complicate up to 46% of cases.

Mortality can be high and confusion with community-acquired pneumonia (CAP) is possible. Like other intracellular diseases interaction between infected host cells and antigen-specific T-cells is integral to cell-mediated immunity (as in TB or leishmaniasis). Occasionally melioidosis may not become apparent for decades after the initial infection. There was an upsurge in reported cases in Sri Lanka after the tsunami of 2004.

Melioidosis is a particular hazard for travellers and military personnel serving overseas. Like Q fever it has also been developed as a potential biological weapon.

28. A. Melioidosis can mimic pulmonary TB, especially in South-East Asia. Many serologically positive people are clinically normal. Overt disease is more likely in those with pre-existing ailments such as diabetes mellitus, renal disease, or immune impairment. Melioidosis is the most common cause of pneumonia in parts of north-east Thailand. Treatment is difficult and prolonged. Ceftazidime and TMP/SMX are preferable to tetracyclines and chloramphenicol.

29. A. Oroya fever is caused by *Bartonella bacilliformis* and is transmitted by phlebotomus sandflies (lutzomyia species). These are night-biters with poor vision and poor powers of flight, seldom moving more than 100 m from their breeding places. Humans are the major reservoir for the disease. Oroya fever is confined to Peru, Bolivia, Colombia, and Ecuador, and is particularly prevalent at altitudes of 600–4000 m. Oroya fever has an incubation period of 6–8 weeks and may cause anaemia, septicaemia, and skin lesions. Sufferers are susceptible to Salmonella infections. Thalassaemia is an abnormality of haemoglobin where there is inability to form one or more of the polypeptide chains. Q fever is transmitted in aerosilized droplets and sometimes by ticks. Plague (*Yersinia pestis*) is transmitted by fleas, usually from infected rats.

30. C. Infected ruminants and cats are the principal reservoirs for *Coxiella burnetti* (*Rickettsia burneti*). It is also carried in rats and other rodents. The infection is maintained in nature by an animal–tick cycle. *C. burnetti* persists in faeces, urine, milk, and other tissues, especially the placenta. Q fever is sometimes a cause of pneumonia in Spain and Portugal.

31. B. A vaccine has been developed in Australia and is useful for those at high risk, e.g. abattoir workers and meat processors. Doxycycline is excellent in acute Q fever. Quinolones or azithromycin are less effective. Acute cases present as fever and pneumonia. In chronic cases, where hepatitis or endocarditis occur, doxycycline together with quinolones or chloroquine for protracted periods is useful. Less than 1% of patients with Q fever die of the condition.

The disease is usually contracted by inhalation of infected aerosols and less commonly by ingestion of raw milk or tick bites. Animal birthing products can swarm with coxiella. The possibility of windborne spread has led to its development as a weapon for biological warfare. Q fever has been notifiable in the USA since 1999. Q fever occurs worldwide.

32. D. The first three are all enteropathogenic protozoa usually transmitted by oocysts which contaminate food or water or are transmitted from person to person. All cause a secretory diarrhoea that is often chronic in nature and may be overwhelming in immunocompromised persons. The bacterium *B. pseudomallei* (melioidosis) is discussed above.

33. Answers: A-3, 6; B-1; C-1; D-3, 5; E-3, 4, 6; F-2

A-3, 6. The itching of onchocerciasis can be absolutely intense, day and night. The itching of scabies ('the itch') is especially severe at night. Insect bites, cercarial dermatitis, larva migrans, superficial fungal infections, and eczema also cause itch.

B-1. Itchy serpentine track-like lesions under the skin are typical of CLM from the hookworm of a dog or cat. These penetrate the bare skin, commonly when walking barefoot. Track-like lesions are also seen in gnathosyomiasis and paragoniasis. The rapid evanescent cutaneous migration of strongyloides (usually on the trunk) only lasts a few days ('larva currens'). Ivermectin (12 mg stat) or albendazole (400 mg every 12 hours for 6 days) are effective in CLM.

C-1. Urticaria can occur whenever helminths are on the move, e.g. in CLM and strongyloides. Urticaria is a non-specific manifestation of acute allergy and is seen also as a response to food additives, contact with allergenic plants, envenomations, and drugs.

D-3, 5. Leishmaniasis is likely to give palpable skin nodules, which are usually found on exposed surfaces and take months to ulcerate. Subcutaneous nodules also occur in onchocerciasis, erythema nodosum, Kaposi sarcoma, and non-tropical conditions such as rheumatoid arthritis and gout.

E-3, 4, 6. Papules are typical of tungiasis (female sandflea, jigger, chigoe flea), which usually occurs near the big toe. They are also seen in many other conditions, including onchocerciasis, scabies, insect bites, and acne.

F-2. Myiasis is an infestation of the skin by the larvae of a diptera fly. See chapter 14.

34. D. Indian Kala-azar ('black sickness') occurs mainly in eastern parts of India, especially in Bihar. It is also endemic in West Bengal and parts of Uttar Pradesh. Sporadic outbreaks occur elsewhere, e.g. Delhi, Jammu, and Kashmir. No animal reservoir exists in India. Both Indian and African varieties are carried by the sandfly. The first VL epidemic in India was reported in 1870.

35. C. PKDL occurs 2–10 years after completion of treatment in 10% of cases in India. It may then last for many years. In contrast PKDL in Africa affects about 3% of patients, comes on quickly, and only lasts a few months. An exception appears to be an outbreak in the Sudan where >50% of treated patients were affected in a mean time of 56 days.

Accessible live parasites (amastigotes) are plentiful in the cutaneous lesions. Although these are non-ulcerative they may be very itchy. HIV patients get a more severe form of PKDL.

36. A. BCG confers protection against leprosy varying from 80% in Uganda to 20% in Myanmar. This is because of cross-reactivity between *M. leprae* and *M. tuberculosis*.

Reflexes are rarely altered in lepromatous neuropathy and this is an important point in diagnosis. The first case of leprosy in a backpacker was reported in 1993 but several other cases have since come to light in non-backpacking short-stay travellers in endemic areas. One such case was reported in a 38-year-old traveller after short stays of <30 days in India, Sri Lanka, and Cuba. Thalidomide is the treatment of choice in erythema nodosum leprosum (ENL), which is a common complication of multibacillary leprosy. It works by acting as an anti-tumour necrosis factor-α (TNF-α), which is grossly elevated in ENL. First-line treatment for leprosy is triple therapy using rifampicin (600 mg/day), clofazimine (50 mg/day), and dapsone (100 mg/day).

37. D. Cutaneous diphtheria is a benign condition which is occasionally imported from developing countries. Diphtheria immunization prevents systemic but not cutaneous diphtheria. Immunization is recommended for travel to Eastern Europe and the Balkans as well as to developing tropical countries.

38. C. Tick paralysis is caused by a neurotoxin injected with the saliva of a tick (*Ixodes holocyclus*). It is common in a 20-km strip on the east coast of Australia but has also been reported elsewhere, e.g. the USA. Removing the tick removes the toxin and full recovery is the rule. The tick often hides in the hair of the host, which is often a child.

39. A. Ascending paralysis similar to that seen in Guillain-Barré syndrome is typical. This contrasts with the descending paralysis of neurotoxic shellfish poisoning and botulism. Initial problems include ataxic gait, multiple rashes, headache, and fever. Respiratory paresis can also occur. The most obvious clue is a history of camping or hiking in tick-infested areas.

40. D. Tick-borne encephalitis virus, which is concentrated in the tick's saliva, passes rapidly into the cells of the skin, although the tick itself may take many days to feed. Tick-borne encephalitis virus is still confined to Europe and Asia but is extending its present geographical habitat.

Tick-borne encephalitis virus is transmitted to humans by ticks, notably *Ixodes ricinus* west of the Urals and *Ixodes persulcatus* east of the Urals. It can also be transmitted orally via unpasteurized milk or cheese from viraemic cattle, goats, and sheep. Tick-borne encephalitis virus is a flavivirus in the same genus as the viruses of yellow fever, dengue fever, Japanese encephalitis and West Nile fever.

41. C. Small rodents are the major reservoir of tick-borne encephalitis virus, with humans an incidental host only. Tick-borne encephalitis virus can survive about 2 hours in acid gastric juice so that active virus can escape to the duodenum and cause disease. Consequently the virus is occasionally contracted by drinking unpasteurized milk. Three subsets of tick-borne encephalitis virus are recognized: European, Siberian, and Far Eastern. The European subtype is clinically far milder than the other two and is often asymptomatic. Carriage of tick-borne encephalitis virus to the CNS across the blood–brain barrier, as with other neurotropic viruses, is probably cytokine enhanced. Some believe such viruses can also be carried directly across by an immune cell (the 'Trojan horse' hypothesis). Note that the adaptive immune system is needed to destroy the tick-borne encephalitis virus antigen and this system is activated by antigen-presenting cells, notably dendritic cells in the skin and gut. Tick saliva contains immunomodulatory substances that affect dendritic cells, thus facilitating the spread of tick-borne encephalitis virus in the body. See question 84 in chapter 2.

42. B. Japanese encephalitis is transmitted by the culicine mosquito, chiefly *Cx. tritaeniorhynchus*, which breeds mainly in rice paddies in rural South-East Asia and the Western Pacific. The virus spreads between birds, especially between wading birds such as herons. Culex transmits it to animals, especially to pigs, which act as amplifying agents. Thereafter it is transmitted to humans, an accidental dead-end host. Japanese encephalitis occurs throughout the year in hot tropical regions but is more seasonal in more moderate northern areas, where epidemics coincide with the monsoons. There is no cure. It is essentially a rural disease, although cases are now occurring in the suburbs of large cities.

43. D. Japanese encephalitis occurs in eastern but not western Russia. Currently Japanese encephalitis is on the increase in the Kathmandu valley and the southern highlands of Nepal. It is hyperendemic in Bali and has been reported in two western tourists who only spent 2 weeks there. It is a year-round hazard in the northern cape of Queensland. Even in Singapore, where it was presumed that Japanese encephalitis was eliminated in the early 1990s, an autochtonous case occurred in 2005. Japanese encephalitis is transmitted to humans by *Ixodes* spp. (ticks).

44. D. Babesiosis is a malaria-like illness that is found only in areas of the USA, Europe, and Asia where the tick vector (*Ixodes* spp.) thrives. Humans are incidental hosts, with cattle, horses, and mice being the primary ones. The first European case was reported in 1957 from Yugoslavia and the first US case, 9 years later, occurred in Nantucket Island. Since then it has been recognized more and more. It is a protozoan infection, which is of serious impact in the elderly and the asplenic. The European variety is often life-threatening and is far more serious than the American one. Fever, chills, and haemolytic anaemia are typical. Treatment is with IV clindamycin and quinine. Babesiosis frequently coexists with Lyme disease.

Respiratory illness, fever, diarrhoea, and dermatitis are the four most frequent medical problems in the returned traveller. Unexplained fever is the most urgent of these because febrile conditions such as malaria, meningitis, and typhoid can all deteriorate rapidly and become life-threatening. Respiratory infections are also very common and are often viral in origin. A persistent cough or a doubtful CXR warrants further investigation.

Diarrhoea that persists may well be helminthic in origin with giardiasis high on the list. In cases already treated with antibiotics one must consider *C. difficile* infection while the unmasking of inflammatory bowel disease or irritable bowel syndrome is probably more common than supposed.

Dermatitis is often due to exacerbation of an existing condition, e.g. psoriasis or eczema. Tropical-related dermatitis is most frequently due to infected arthropod bites. CLM is the main parasitic cause.

Exanthems and enanthems occur in a variety of systemic conditions ranging from acute HIV to dengue fever to coxsackie infection. Rashes are seldom diagnostic unless the cause is obvious, e.g. scabies or typhoid (rose spots).

In all cases the practitioner should adhere to a strict protocol that involves a good history, careful physical examination, and routine screening and microscopy of blood, urine, and stool. Simple X-rays and ultrasound examination may also be considered. In no case should the practitioner hesitate to refer the patient to a specialist physician.

Nowadays computer-assisted diagnosis is becoming more popular and more reliable. The Kabisa Travel System, developed in Antwerp, has been shown to perform equally well with travel physicians in diagnosing the cause of fever in those returned from a tropical environment. Kabisa is the Swaili word for 'hand in the fire, I am absolutely certain'!

1. **What is the treatment for an adult patient who has brucellosis?**
    A. Co-trimoxazole 800 mg bid × 4–6 weeks
    B. Rifampicin 600–900 mg daily × 4–6 weeks
    C. Doxycycline 100 mg bid × 4–6 weeks
    D. Doxycycline as above plus another antibiotic, e.g. streptomycin, × 2–3 weeks

2. **A traveller from the Central Pacific with acute LF is likely to show**
   A. Diurnal microfilaraemia
   B. Nocturnal microfilaraemia
   C. Microfilaraemia at any time
   D. Marked eosinophilia at night

3. **A traveller has been home for 6 months from a short visit to Ghana. She now has non-itchy migratory swellings in the calves, forearms, and wrists that last for a few days at a time. Which is the most likely diagnosis?**
   A. CLM
   B. Loa loa
   C. Allergy to her antimalarial prophylactics
   D. Migrating allergy to the jigger worm

4. **Which of these is the most suggestive of acute leptospirosis in a febrile traveller from an endemic area?**
   A. Headache
   B. Jaundice
   C. Rash on the extremities
   D. Conjunctival suffusion

5. **A 35-year-old male is 1 week back from a 2-month trip to Thailand. He has fever (37.8°C), vomiting, diarrhoea, and oliguria (<800 ml/day). His white blood cell count is 14,000/mm³. Serum creatinine is 68 μmol/l. He is probably suffering from**
   A. Malaria
   B. Gastroenteritis
   C. Leptospirosis
   D. Hantavirus

6. **A 30-year-old traveller is 5 days back from a package holiday to Turkey. He now complains of nausea, vomiting, explosive watery foul-smelling diarrhoea, sulphurous belching, and abdominal distension. The most likely diagnosis is**
   A. Giardiasis
   B. *E. coli* enteritis
   C. Rotavirus infection
   D. Acute salmonellosis

7. A 40-year-old woman has just returned from 7 weeks in Pakistan where she was an administrator in a small **NGO** working in areas devastated by landslides. She says that within 6 hours of eating a meal 'in the field' she felt her 'tummy in knots'. Since then she has had flatulence, passes foul-smelling greasy stools about three times a day, and on occasion has felt her abdomen swelling. She took local homeopathic medicine and cefeximine (semisynthetic cephalosporin) with little benefit. She is afebrile and has no obvious blood in her stool. You firstly suspect
    A. *E. coli* diarrhoea
    B. Tropical sprue
    C. Cryptosporidiosis
    D. Giardiasis

8. **Which of the following do you consider most typical of Katayama syndrome (acute schistosomiasis)?**
    A. Hepatosplenomegaly
    B. Itchy rash
    C. Decreased platelet count
    D. Eosinophilia

9. **Acute schistosomiasis (Katayama fever)**
    A. Is strongly associated with *S. mekongi* infection
    B. Is closely correlated with the intensity of the schistosomal infection
    C. Is an important cause of fever in immigrants from endemic areas
    D. Is virtually confined to exposed non-immune travellers

10. **The diagnosis of schistosomiasis in travelers is usually made by**
    A. Finding cercariae in the blood
    B. Serological antibody assays
    C. The appearance of typical eggs in the urine or faeces from the second week after infection
    D. Early hepatic enlargement

11. **When treating schistosomiasis**
    A. Avoid PZQ in pregnancy
    B. Avoid PZQ in small children
    C. Use PZQ as early as possible after exposure so that the disease may be aborted
    D. Use corticosteroids in acute schistosomiasis (Katayama fever)

12. **An asymptomatic traveller is 2 weeks back from Rwanda and confesses that he swam frequently in Lake Muhazi during the last month. He is worried that he may have contracted schistosomiasis. Should you**

    A. Give PZQ in appropriate dosage (40 mg/kg)
    B. Reassure him that he is safe at the moment but ask him to return for serology in 3 months
    C. Test for serum antibodies against schistosome (adult worm and/or egg)
    D. Wait until symptoms suggestive of Katayama fever appear before starting treatment

13. **A 22-year-old man has returned from a 6-month stay in Mali. He took chloroquin and proguanil irregularly for malarial prophylaxis, swam in a local waterfall, had several unprotected sexual contacts, and lived for a month in an inland village. Apart from a few bouts of diarrhoea and one attack of self-diagnosed malaria for which he took co-arthemeter, he was well while overseas. A week after returning to Europe he developed some testicular pain and said his ejaculate was less viscous and darker in colour than usual. Your most likely diagnosis is**

    A. Tuberculosis
    B. Schistosomiasis
    C. Drug reaction
    D. Seminoma of the testis

14. **A middle-aged missionary who has worked for many years in Turkana (northern Kenya) is home on leave and complains of progressive loss of weight and intermittent fever for the past 6 months. However, he feels well although he looks very pale. Examination reveals a smooth, greatly enlarged liver, an easily palpable spleen, and generalized lymphadenopathy. There is anaemia and leucopenia. In view of the circumstances you are most suspicious of**

    A. Hydatid disease
    B. Visceral leishmaniasis
    C. Cysticercosis
    D. Hepatoma

15. **How would you best confirm your diagnosis in the above case?**

    A. Do three blood films for parasites
    B. Examine for Leishman–Donovan bodies in aspirate (spleen, bone marrow, lymph nodes)
    C. Serology for parasite antibodies
    D. Positive leishmanin skin test

16. **Match the diseases with the most likely history. Items 1, 2, 3, and 4 can be used once, more than once, or not at all**

    A. Schistosomiasis
    B. Leptospirosis
    C. HIV
    D. Brucellosis
    E. Tuberculosis
    F. Hepatitis B

    1. White water rafting
    2. Received tattoo while abroad
    3. Skin contact with fresh or brackish water
    4. Consumed raw dairy products

17. **Match a disease with one of the following symptoms/signs. Items A, B, C, and D can be used once, more than once, or not at all**

    A. Viral hepatitis
    B. Dengue fever
    C. Rickettsiosis
    D. Tropical pulmonary eosinophilia
    E. Diphtheria
    F. Malaria

    1. Maculopapular rash
    2. Cough or dyspnea
    3. Jaundice
    4. Sore throat

18. **Those with fever and haemorrhagic signs who have returned from a country where VHF has been reported in the last 5 years should be isolated**

    A. If they have returned in the last 3 weeks
    B. If they have returned in the last 3 months
    C. If they have returned in the last year but have worked in a hospital overseas
    D. If they show signs of neurological or respiratory distress irrespective of how long they are home

19. **A febrile backpacker is 1 week back from Malawi. He admits to swimming on one occasion in lake Malawi 4 weeks ago. Physical examination is normal. His full blood count is normal. The most likely diagnosis is**

    A. Malaria
    B. Schistosomiasis (Katayama fever)
    C. Acute HIV
    D. Non-specific viral infection

20. **A traveller is 5 days home from the Serengeti. He has a 'chancre' on his forearm where he has been bitten by a 'bug'. It is red, indurated, and painful. He has now developed a high fever, headache, and signs of meningism. He has had all the correct immunizations and has taken mefloquine regularly. He is most likely to have**

    A. Malaria
    B. Leishmaniasis
    C. Trypanosomiasis
    D. Dengue fever

21. **A 10-year-old develops the following within 6 weeks of returning home to Europe from Bangladesh, where he stayed with his relatives for 2 months: abdominal pain, diarrhoea, high fever, severe headache, and a few pink macules on his chest. He has relative bradycardia and a blood count shows moderate leucopenia. What is the most likely diagnosis?**
    A. Meningitis
    B. Salmonellosis
    C. Typhoid fever
    D. Malaria

22. **Which of the following is most likely in a man just back from India who has abdominal pain, moderate diarrhoea, and high fever with a leucocyte count <8000/ml?**
    A. Amoebic liver abscess
    B. Typhoid fever
    C. Non-typhoid gastroenteritis
    D. Acute Crohn's disease

23. **Which of the following is the most suggestive of acute HIV in a high-risk febrile traveller?**
    A. Lymphadenopathy
    B. Palatal enathem
    C. Leucopenia
    D. Thrombocytopenia.

24. **A fully immunized 65-year-old man is just back from a month's shooting holiday in Zimbabwe. Two weeks into his holiday he developed 'flu like symptoms, a mild fever, and a rash all over his trunk. He now feels 'out of sorts'. He says many of his party got tick bites but not him. There is no abnormality on physical examination. What do you suspect?**
    A. Malaria
    B. Rickettsia
    C. Schistosomiasis
    D. Leishmaniasis

25. **A frequent business visitor to China presents with fever, chills, and headache 3 months after returning from his last visit. Clinical examination is normal except for mild tenderness in the left hypochondrium. Blood reports include WBC 2000 cells/mm³, Hb 15.5 g/dl, and platelets 55,000/mm³. Malaria smears are negative as is dengue serology, including the NS1 dengue test. Splenomegaly is shown on abdominal imaging. The patient took atovaquone/proguanil (Malarone™) conscientiously on every trip, ate carefully, and merely commuted from hotel to work and back. After 2 weeks of multiple antibiotic therapy there was no improvement. Select one of the following as the most likely diagnosis**

    A. Typhoid fever
    B. Malaria
    C. Dengue fever
    D. Leptospirosis

26. **First-time acute phase infections are associated initially with a rise in**

    A. IgG
    B. IgA
    C. IgM
    D. IgE

27. **False positive serology (raised IgG) in a patient with dengue fever may occur in travellers who have been previously vaccinated against**

    A. Polio (oral)
    B. Japanese encephalitis virus
    C. Chikungunya
    D. Rubella

28. **A 35-year-old male is 2 years home from Iraq where he served with the armed forces. While there he had at least two bouts of diarrhoea, one of which was bloody. He now has a high swinging fever, tender palpable liver, and a moderate leucocytosis. Which of the following would you do first in order to arrive at a quick diagnosis?**

    A. Liver function tests
    B. Blood culture
    C. Liver ultrasound
    D. C reactive protein

29. **Which of the following do you consider to be the most likely diagnosis in question 28?**
    A. Pyogenic liver abscess
    B. Amoebic liver abscess
    C. Infected hydatid cyst
    D. Acute hepatoma

30. **A businessman has returned to the USA after a year in China. He has moderate fever and abdominal discomfort. On examination he has definite hepatomegaly. He has a marked eosinophilia. If you could only do one of the following investigations initially, which would you choose?**
    A. Serology for hepatitis
    B. Ultrasound of the liver
    C. CXR
    D. Stools for culture, ova, and parasites

31. **You have out-ruled amoebiasis in the above patient. Which of the following is the most likely?**
    A. Recurrent malaria
    B. Liver fluke
    C. Visceral leishmaniasis
    D. Viral hepatitis

32. **A 40-year-old woman from Kazakhstan (Central Asia) has lived in Europe for the past 6 years. She now complains of intermittent right upper abdominal pain that lasts only a few hours, progressive loss of weight, anorexia, lassitude, and occasional fever. When in Kazakhstan she worked in a nuclear plant and ate regularly in the canteen. Fish from Lake Balkhash was frequently on the menu. A likely diagnosis is**
    A. Gall stones
    B. Hepatitis A
    C. Hepatitis C
    D. Oriental liver fluke

33. **What treatment would you give the woman in question 32?**
    A. Albendazole (prolonged course)
    B. Doxycycline (minimum 10 days)
    C. Metronidazole or tinidazole (minimum 10 days)
    D. PZQ

34. **An otherwise healthy 40-year-old man complains of sudden severe headaches associated with vomiting about 1 month after returning from a trip to Korea where he attended a wedding and ate the local food. CNS examination is normal. Which of the tests below is the most appropriate initially?**

    A. MRI scan
    B. Lumbar puncture
    C. Blood culture
    D. BP monitoring during headaches

35. **A lumbar puncture in the above case shows a mild increase in intracranial pressure and many eosinophils in the CSF. Which of the following do you most suspect?**

    A. Typhoid
    B. Neural schistosomiasis
    C. *Angiostrongylus cantonensis* (rat lungworm)
    D. *Gnathosyomiasis spinigerum*

36. **A 32-year-old Australian diplomat based in Korea has spent his holidays for the last 5 years travelling in the Far East and South-East Asia. He now complains of cough and the regular expectoration of discoloured sputum, which on at least five occasions contained dark staining material that he thinks was blood. Despite all pertinent vaccinations he has had bouts of fever, diarrhoea, and abdominal pain from time to time, which he put down to dietary indiscretion. He admits to have eaten local food regularly, including seafood soaked in vinegar or wine. He has a marked eosinophilia. CXR shows mottling in both apices and a cavity in the left mid zone. His tuberculin test (TT) is negative. He is likely to be suffering from**

    A. Tuberculosis
    B. Paragonia
    C. Melioidosis
    D. Tropical pulmonary eosinophilia (TPE)

37. **A 38-year-old career aid worker is back from Ecuador having spent 10 years there. A month after returning to Canada she suddenly developed a grand mal seizure. This was repeated a week later. There are several palpable, movable, painless subcutaneous nodules each 1–2 cm in size on her back. CXR, full blood count, fasting blood sugar, urine, and CSF are normal. There is no family history of epilepsy. Which of the following is the most likely?**

    A. Neurocystisercosis
    B. Tuberculoma
    C. Brain tumour
    D. Late onset epilepsy

38. **How do you best treat cysticercosis?**
    A. Emetine
    B. Metronidazole
    C. PZQ
    D. Ivermectin

39. **An AIDS patient who is on HAART but not on prophylaxis against** *P. jirovecii* **returns from the tropics with a prolonged profuse watery diarrhoea. He is most likely to have**
    A. *Cyclospora cayetanensis*
    B. Giardiasis
    C. Amoebiasis
    D. Cholera

40. **A 40-year-old man is just back from Thailand after a 2-week business trip. He has a urethral discharge and dysuria for 2 days. On examination he has a few small painful shallow ulcers on the corona of his penis. He denies sexual contact in Thailand. He admits bathing once in the Mekong delta area during an outing from work. Which of the following do you consider most likely?**
    A. Schistosomiasis
    B. Lymphogranuloma venerum
    C. Gonorrhea
    D. HIV

41. **What further steps would you take in the case of 40?**
    A. Warn his wife/partner in confidence
    B. Screen blood for other STIs
    C. Trace and treat contacts
    D. Advise counselling

42. **An ulcerative skin lesion <2.5 cm in diameter on the forearm of a traveller recently home from Kenya is most likely**
    A. Anthrax
    B. Cutaneous leishmaniasis
    C. A septic insect bite
    D. Rickettsial eschar

43. **An isolated eosinophilia of >500/mm³ in a long-term traveller returned from the developing world should lead to a suspicion of**
    A. Strongyloides
    B. Chronic malaria
    C. Dengue fever
    D. Rickettsia

44. **A traveller receiving daily corticosteroids for rheumatoid arthritis is 8 weeks back from South-East Asia where he had spent 3 months involved in construction work. Apart from a few bouts of diarrhoea he has been well. He is now complaining of weight loss, vague abdominal pain, occasional diarrhoea, and an irritating cough and wheeze which is made worse by smoking. Which of the following is the most likely cause?**
    A. Opisthorchiasis (clonorchiasis)
    B. Giardiasis
    C. Strongyloides
    D. Amoebiasis

45. **Which is the most useful investigation in confirming the diagnosis of strongyloides?**
    A. Stool samples for the larvae of S. *stercoralis*
    B. Differential white cell count
    C. D-xylose absorption test
    D. ELISA serology for antibodies

46. **A 26-year-old traveller is a week home in London after spending 2 weeks in July in the Algarve (southern Portugal). He has been bitten several times by mosquitoes. He complains of headache, fever, and mild photophobia. Which of the following is most likely?**
    A. Malaria
    B. West Nile fever
    C. Meningitis
    D. Dengue fever

47. **What is the best way to diagnose suspected WNV infection in someone just back from an endemic area?**
    A. A history of visiting an endemic area
    B. Do specific IgG levels in the plasma
    C. Do specific IgM levels in plasma
    D. Blood culture

48. **A Peace Corps worker is 2 years back from West Africa. He has itching of the eyes and skin. What do you suspect most?**
    A. Scabies
    B. Onchocerciasis
    C. CLM
    D. Strongyloides

49. **How long after infection might you identify onchocercal microfilariae in skin snips?**
    A. 1–3 weeks
    B. 1–3 months
    C. 3–6 months
    D. 10–30 months

50. **A 21-year-old medical student is doing an elective in Malawi and, while assisting at a Caesarean section on a 16-year-old primagravida, sustains a needle stick injury in her thumb. She phones you for advice. Should she**
    A. Not worry if the patient's blood proves HIV negative
    B. Start HAART immediately and finish her elective stint in Malawi
    C. Start antiretrovirals and come home immediately
    D. Make sure she has had a tetanus shot and check her HIV status in 6 weeks

51. **A 33-year-old woman from South America was admitted to Nsambya hospital, Kampala, complaining of persistent vomiting and loss of weight. Blood, urine, and stool examination was normal, as was physical examination. Barium studies revealed a smoothly constricted lower end of the oesophagus. Which of these is highest on your list of possibilities?**
    A. Cancer of the oesophagus
    B. Chagas' disease
    C. Primary achalasia
    D. Hysteria

52. **A long-term expatriate complains that food 'sticks in my chest' after swallowing. He also complains that 'sometimes my mouth is sore'. On examination there are some small ulcers around the corners of the mouth and a few white plaques inside the cheeks which scrape off easily. He is most likely to have**
    A. Candida infection
    B. Oral herpes
    C. Kaposi sarcoma
    D. Leukoplakia

53. **Infection with the soil fungus *Fusarium dimerum* should be strongly suspected in an immunocompromised person who has spent a month in a rural setting and who presents with**
    A. Sudden onset of fever and joint pain
    B. Eye pain
    C. Ataxic gait
    D. Mildly pruritic rash on arms and trunk

1. D. Double or, in severe cases, triple therapy for a prolonged period is always recommended. In pregnancy one can use rifampicin plus co-trimoxazole.

2. A. Daytime microfilaraemia coinciding with daytime mosquto bites occurs in about 70% of those with acute LF from the Central Pacific. As in other helminthic conditions an eosinophilia (day and night) is likely to be present. Nocturnal microfilaraemia is the rule with night biting vectors, e.g. with *W. bancrofti* in Africa. Microflaraemia is less commonly found in travellers with chronic LF.

3. B. These migrating oedematous areas are typical 'Calabar swellings' associated with an allergic response to migration of the adult filarial worm of loa loa. The swellings last about 3 days and are mildly itchy. Sheathed microfilaria may appear in the peripheral blood during the day (1000–1500 hours). The vector is the large red crysops fly that infects the forest canopy in West Africa and lays its eggs in slow-moving muddy water. Loias is found only in Africa where it occurs from the Gulf of Guinea to the Great Central African lakes. It is best known for the subconjunctival migration of the adult worm (<7 cm). This causes itchiness, redness, and pain in the affected eye but also affords an ideal chance to remove the parasite.

CLM is intensely itchy and can be seen as a migrating serpiginous coil under the skin.

Allergies to antimalarials appear while the traveller is taking them and usually are manifest as a generalized itchy rash.

The jigger flea (chigoe flea, tungiasis) is typically confined to the feet or lower legs, and has a brown central area representing the gravid female.

4. D. Conjunctival suffusion occurs in over 50% of patients with leptospirosis. Mild hepatorenal dysfunction often occurs and may be severe in overt Weils disease (*L. icterohemorrhagica*). If a rash occurs in leptospirosis it is mainly on the trunk. A history of exposure is a key factor in making the diagnosis.

5. C. Leptospirosis has manifestations varying from a mild illness to Weils disease. The sudden onset of a febrile illness with chills, abdominal pain, myalgia, headache, conjunctival suffusion (not found in the above case), and skin rash is frequently found. Some renal impairment occurs in 45–65% of patients and gastrointestinal symptoms are also common (10–30%).

Leptospirosis is on the increase in Thailand, more so since the tsunami struck. It is contracted by contact with water that is contaminated by urine from infected animals, usually rats.

Malaria should be excluded as a routine. Occasionally gastroenteritis due to *E. coli* O157 or hantavirus infection is associated with similar symptoms.

6. A. Giardiasis is typically associated with these symptoms. Diagnosis depends on identifying the cysts in one or more fresh or properly preserved stools. Tests for parasite antigen in the stool are probably just as good but may give false negative results. The cysts look remarkably like little faces, hence the connotation 'faces in the faeces'.

7. D. These findings are again typical of giardiasis. Frequently patients can pinpoint the meal at which they acquired the infection. In this case fresh stools teemed with typical trophozoites. Treatment with metronidazole 400 mg three times a day for 5 days cured the patient. Tinidazole 2 g in divided doses for adults and 50 mg/kg for children is preferable but more expensive. Albendazole 400 mg daily for 5 days is also effective. Giardiasis is the most common cause of protozoan post-travel diarrhoea. It is found worldwide but is extremely common in situations where hygiene is poor and there is a lack of proper infrastructure.

8. D. Eosinophilia and urticaria are most typical. Fever, rash, diarrhoea, cough, and hepatosplenomegaly also occur. The initial cercarial dermatitis is not to be confused with Katayama fever, which appears later. It is a popular misconception that initial cercarial dermatitis (swimmer's itch) is always a feature of schistosomal infection in non-immune travellers. Schistosomiasis is also known as bilharziasis after Theodor Bilharz, who first described the parasite in urinary disease in 1851. The full disease cycle was not described until 1908 by Piraja da Silva.

9. D. Katayama fever is almost unknown in immigrants and rarely occurs in local populations where repeated exposure from before birth, and increasing worm load as the individual matures, lead to a gradual accommodation by the host so that the person is either asymptomatic or else presents de novo with classical chronic schistosomiasis. Katayama fever is far more likely to occur in non-immune travellers, where it is responsible for 2–4% of cases of fever.

There is almost always a history of contact with fresh water in endemic areas such as the great lakes in Central Africa, the Dogon valley, and Volta lake in West Africa, Lake Muhazi (Rwanda), Lake Malawi, and Lake Victoria. It is believed that Katayama fever is due to a hypersensitive reaction to schistosomules that have matured in the liver and are now exiting from that organ. It generally occurs about 4 weeks after exposure to the infection. Katayama fever is mostly confined to S. haematobium and S. mansoni but, should it occur after S. japonicum, it may persist and evolve into severe hepatic fibrosis and portal hypertension. The name 'Katayama' comes from the Katayama region near Hiroshima in Japan where the condition was first described as a response to S. japonicum.

10. B. Serum antibody assays are sensitive but cannot distinguish active from past infection. Thus they are of limited value in evaluating immigrants and asylum seekers. Nonetheless they are useful in the case of travellers who have been to endemic areas, are home some months, and complain of vague symptoms such as depression which you cannot ascribe to another disease.

Microhaematuria and microscopy of urinary sediment for erythrocytes is a useful adjunct in the diagnosis of S. haematobium if serology is even weakly positive. Eggs may not be found at any stage and do not appear in the urine or faeces before 4 weeks. If present they have a typical appearance. Hypereosinophilia (>1000 µl^{-1}) is common but not invariable in Katayama fever. Nonetheless an eosinophilia or an elevated IgE are useful adjuncts in making the diagnosis. Diagnosis largely depends on a history of exposure to infected water, an option not mentioned above.

11. D. Steroids suppress the inflammatory/hypersensitivity reaction to the schistosomal antigen both in Katayama fever and in neuroschistosomiasis and should be used in conjunction with PZQ in both situations. Larger than usual doses of steroids may be used because steroids can reduce the plasma level of PZQ by as much as 50%. Steroids should never be given if there is coexistent strongyloides for fear of disseminating this condition. Normally one adds anticonvulsants in neuroschistosomiasis, especially where there is transverse myelitis.

PZQ appears to be safe to use both in pregnancy and in small children. PZQ treatment should be delayed at least 4 weeks after exposure to the disease since it only affects schistosomules after they have matured in the liver.

12. B. In relation to exposure, the mean time for serology to become positive is 5–10 weeks or longer, as documented in a group of Belgians who had merely paddled in Lake Muhazi. In relation to symptoms, seroconversion does not occur until 2 weeks after the clinical signs of Katayama fever. This means that you cannot normally diagnose the condition with certainty for some months. Furthermore, although Katayama fever is very common in infected Western travellers, it is rare in those brought up in endemic areas.

13. B. Schistosomiasis, especially *S. hematobium*, is endemic in Mali and several cases have been reported in travellers to that country, especially in those who came into contact with waterfalls in Dogon. Haemospermia and changes in the colour and viscosity of ejaculate are typical. The female schistosome lays eggs in the hypogastric plexus and these subsequently appear in any part of the genitourinary tract or rectum depending on the species involved. Genitourinary TB may present with painless haematuria but is unlikely because symptoms appeared within a week of the patient returning to Europe. There have been no such symptoms reported after chloroquine/proguanil or co-arthemeter. A seminoma, most common in men in their 40s, usually presents as a progressive painless tumour of the testis which may reach ten times its normal size. Sometimes a hydrocoel obscures the testicular swelling, rarely the testis is painful. An STI is likely to present with urethral discharge, penile ulceration, and frequently pain on urination.

14. B. Visceral leishmaniasis (kala azar) is characterized by all these findings. The spleen and liver sometimes attain a very large size. Infection is via the bite of an infected female sandfly and while most cases occur in the Indian subcontinent it is also common in Sudan and Turkana (*L. donovani* and *L. tropica*). Hydatid disease is caused by ingestion of ova of *Echinococcus granulosus*, the dog tapeworm. Turkana probably has more cases per person than any other area of the world due to the close association of human and canine populations and poor hygiene. The cysts occur in the liver (70%), lungs (20%), and elsewhere. Clearly it must also be considered in this case. Cysticercosis is due to ingestion of ova of *Taenia solium* and is characterized by multiple painless subcutaneous cysts or less commonly by cysts in muscle and brain (see below). Hepatoma is an aggressive tumour of the liver likely to occur in those with chronic hepatitis B in which the palpable liver is hard and nodular. Ascites may be present. Chronic malaria is more often associated with splenomegaly. When hepatomegaly occurs it is seldom to the extent found in this patient. Nor does the adenopathy fit this diagnosis. Advanced lymphoma is a possibility but the fact that the patient feels so well is against this diagnosis.

15. B. Splenic aspiration may reveal scanty Leishman–Donovan bodies (amastigotes) in >95% of cases. Aspirates from bone marrow (>85%), buffy coat (>70%), and lymph nodes (>65%) are also useful. Amastigotes may be detected in peripheral blood in about 50% of HIV-associated cases. Urine or serum antigen tests are also useful but not as definite as amastigote identification. The leishmanin skin test (Montenegro test), in which killed promastigotes are injected intradermally and the resulting reaction 'read' in 48 hours, is often negative in VL, although it may become positive after successful treatment.

16. Answers: A-1, 3; B-1, 3; C-2; D-4; E-4; F-2.

17. Answers: A-3; B-1; C-1; D-2, 4; E-4; F-2.

18. A. The incubation period of the serious VHFs is less than 3 weeks. Isolation is expensive and time-consuming, and reference should be made to the region of travel: Crimean-Congo fever (Asia, Eastern Europe, all Africa excluding North Africa), Lassa fever (rural West Africa), ebola (Sudan, Congo, Uganda, Kenya), marburg (widespread). Note that we exclude non-contagious VHFs such as dengue fever. In practice the incubation period of VHFs is <14 days. Recent outbreaks of ebola and yellow fever in Uganda within 50 miles of Kampala are a cause for concern to travellers.

19. A. Malaria is the most likely diagnosis and is of immediate concern. One also considers Katayama fever (of which fever may be the only sign) but this is unlikely because of the absence of an eosinophilia or rash. Acute HIV can present with fever, adenitis, and pharyngitis but fever alone is rare. Other viral fevers usually present with fever, headache, myalgia, arthralgia, and general malaise.

20. C. Exposure to the tsetse fly in the bush or woodlands of East Africa can cause infection with *Trypanosoma rhodesiense*. Although the risk is small in travellers it seems to be increasing. Tsetse flies bite during the day and are attracted by dark colours, contrasting colours, and moving vehicles. Metacyclic trypanosomes multiply at the site of inoculation before entering the blood to disseminate widely as trypomastigotes. A chancre usually appears 2–3 days after the bite and fever begins 1–3 weeks later. Trypanosomes may be seen in thick blood films. Arsenic-based drugs are still the mainstay of treatment. African leishmaniasis (carried by sandflies) is much slower to develop. Malaria is very unlikely if the patient is on mefloquine and dengue fever is rare in travellers to East Africa.

21. C. While all of the options enter the differential diagnosis the most likely cause of the child's illness is *S. typhi*. *S. typhi* has an incubation period of 3–60 days, with 'typical' cases having an incubation period of 8–18 days. Diarrhoea is more common than constipation and 'rose spots' (2–5 mm macules that fade on pressure) are uncommon.

A positive culture from bone marrow (the best site), blood, stool, or urine is the only certain way to diagnose typhoid fever. The much denigrated Widal test can also be helpful when interpreted thoughtfully.

In general antibiotics such as third-generation cephalosporins, e.g. ceftriaxone, the fluorquinolones, or azithromycin, are very effective. Note, however, the recent rise in quinolone resistance.

Those who visit friends and relatives in developing countries are often under the illusion that they have immunity to any disease they may encounter during their holiday and often take risks that other travellers will not take. While adults born overseas may have residual immunity, their children born in the West will have none whatsoever.

22. B. Typhoid fever is the prime suspect given the location of the travel and the findings listed. After collecting stool, urine, and blood for culture, anti-typhoid treatment should be started.

Always outrule coexistent malaria unless you are certain the traveller has only visited areas below 2500 m. Amoebic abscess is a possibility but there will be tenderness in the right hypochondrium and usually a significant leucocytosis (>10,000/ml). Liver ultrasound is useful in locating an abscess. Serology is >90% sensitive in the diagnosis of amoebiasis but it should be noted that many patients cannot recall having had dysentery.

Non-typhoid gastroenteritis will respond to the antibiotics used against *S. typhi*. Finally bear in mind the possibility of an acute abdomen.

23. B. Acute seroconversion illness depends on a history of exposure to infected body fluids but this history is not always forthcoming. While all or any of the options listed may be found, palatal reddening is probably the most suggestive of acute HIV in the traveller.

24. B. A diagnosis of African tick bite fever is justified. The condition is widespread in Zimbabwe and southern Africa, where it is usually caused by *R. conorii*, although in Zimbabwe it is more likely to be *R. africae*. It has a short incubation period and is readily cured by doxycycline. This case was unusual in that no eschar was remembered and despite other members of his party complaining of tick bites this patient did not notice any.

Domestic cattle, rhinoceros, and hippopotamus form a natural reservoir for *R. conorii* and *R. africae* in the veldt and grasslands (personal case).

25. B. This patient had *P. ovale* malaria in which the hypnozoites reactivated the disease once primary prophylaxis with malarone was over. Treatment with 15–30 mg primaquine daily for 14 days cured him. Two weeks terminal prophylaxis with primaquine is recommended for all those who spend long periods (or recurrent shorter periods) in endemic areas provided the G6PD test is normal and the patient is neither pregnant nor nursing. The CDC recommends primaquine to such persons –1 to +7 days (similar to malarone schedule). Options A, C, and D are all possible but less likely in view of his history and his failure to respond to antibiotics.

26. C. IgM appears first and this is followed later by the more specific IgG. The spleen is important in producing IgM against encapsulated organisms and parasites.

27. B. Serological cross-reactivity can occur with other flaviviruses, e.g. Japanese encephalitis, tick-borne encephalitis, yellow fever, and dengue fever.

28. C. Clearly we can include all the options as part of a general work up. However, in this case we expect liver function tests to be abnormal and the acute phase proteins to be elevated so that these tests hardly further the diagnosis. Blood culture will take some days to interpret but we want to arrive at a diagnosis as soon as possible, thus liver ultrasound is a sensible immediate choice since it can show cysts and tumours, and distinguish true hepatomegaly from a spurious one due to pulmonary pathology, e.g. pleural effusion. It is also cheap, quick, non–invasive, and easily accessible.

29. B. An amoebic liver abscess should be suspected in anyone who has lived in an endemic area, particularly with a history of diarrhoea/dysentery. Often an amoebic liver abscess will not present for several years after the initial infection and a history of diarrhoea may be lacking. Treat with metronidazole 800 mg tid × 7 days or tinidazole 2 g daily for 5 days.

A pyogenic abscess is unusual and either comes from a nearby source, e.g. pneumonia, or via an infected embolus in a patient with ulcerative colitis or Crohn's disease. A marked leucocytosis would be expected. Eighty per cent of hydatid cysts (*E. granulosus*) occur in the liver and are usually silent until they rupture with signs of shock and collapse. Small leaks are associated with urticaria, pruritus, and jaundice. Hydatid liver disease is diagnosed by sonography and confirmed by serology, which has replaced the old Casoni test. Be sure to distinguish between amoebic liver cysts and dog tapeworm (hydatid) cysts.

30. B. Liver imaging should be done folowed by serology for amoebiasis. If these tests are negative proceed with the other options. Amoebic liver abscess is the most urgent item to consider because of the danger of rupture into the pleural or peritoneal cavities.

31. B. It is likely that this patient has a local liver fluke, e.g. *Opisthorchiasis* (syn. *Clonorchis*) *sinensis* or *O. viverreni*. These are contracted by eating undercooked fish or meat or even from using contaminated utensils in China or South-East Asia. *O. viverrini* is the most common cause of liver cancer in north-east Thailand.

Recurrent malaria can also present with fever and hepatomegaly. However, eosinophilia is not the rule unless there is coexistent helminthiasis, although eosinophilia has been reported in helminth-free Thai patients 6 weeks after *P. falciparum* has been cleared from the blood. Visceral leishmaniasis is not to be expected in a visiting businessman, but splenomegaly is more typical of VL and this was not present in this patient. One expects a businessman to have been vaccinated against hepatitis A and B. Nonetheless serology for HAV, HBV, and HEV should also be performed.

32. D. *Opisthorchis felineus* is the type of liver fluke most common in Russia and Eastern Europe. Eggs are passed in the faeces of humans and animals (especially dogs and cats), and eventually humans consume the metacercariae in contaminated raw or undercooked fish or from poorly washed utensils, as with the Chinese fluke (above). Recurrent bouts of ascending cholangitis occur and gallstones may be suspected or may occur concomitantly. Jaundice occurs in serious cases. Untreated the condition may cause cholangiocarcinoma. Neither hepatitis A nor hepatitis C cause short recurrent bouts of cholangitis. In cholelithiasis gall bladder colic is prominent (personal case).

33. D. The treatment of choice for oriental liver fluke is PZQ 40 mg/kg as a stat dose or in two divided doses 4–6 hours apart or in a lower dose of 25 mg/kg tid for 3 days. Higher and repeated doses are given in heavy infestation.

Albendazole is used in hydatid disease, CLM, and strongyloides, while metronidazole or tinidazole is used in hookworm and amoebiasis. Note that PZQ is unreliable for treating liver fluke due to *Fascioliasis*. This liver fluke is common in cattle- and sheep-rearing areas, especially in Peru and Bolivia, and should be treated with bithionol or nitazoxanide.

34. B. This man appears to have the symptoms of mildly raised intracranial pressure (ICP). A CT brain scan should confirm or outrule this. If the ICP is not markedly elevated then a lumbar puncture can be done and the CSF sent for culture, cytology, and routine examination, e.g. protein, differential white cell count, and glucose concentration.

35. C. *A. cantonensis* is endemic in China, Korea, South-East Asia, and the South Pacific, where consumption of raw fish is common. Raw snails (a delicacy often given at celebrations such as weddings), raw or undercooked fish, or raw vegetables contaminated with the parasite are usually implicated. *A. cantonensis* is deposited in rat's faeces and eaten by slugs and snails (which humans eat) or it may contaminate fish or vegetables, which are ingested by humans.

In humans the larvae penetrate the intestinal mucosa and enter the CNS where, in the course of 5–8 weeks, they die. Mostly they cause no ill-effects but sometimes they cause CNS symptoms and present as an EM. Steroids seem to be the only therapy that helps.

G. spinigerum in the CNS causes a stormier disease with obvious palsies and sensory damage, while neural schistosomiasis generally affects the conus medullaris.

Typhoid fever will exhibit the features of fever, abdominal discomfort, and altered bowel habit. Bone marrow/blood/urine culture will be positive for *S. typhi*.

36. B. A history of having eaten uncooked crabs or crayfish soaked in brine, wine, alcohol, or vinegar in the Far East together with haemoptysis and eosinophilia is characteristic of infection with the lung fluke *Paragonimus westermani*. *P. westermani* (Oriental lung fluke) is the most common of the 10 species of paragonia known to infect humans. This condition also occurs focally in West Africa, parts of north-west South America, and northern India.

The life cycle involves ingestion of pickled crabs and crayfish that contain the metacercariae of the fluke. Once in the human duodenum the parasite travels to the lungs, where it causes abscess and cavity formation with haemoptysis. Chronic cough, loss of weight, and superinfection are typical. Subsequent contamination of ponds or rivers by eggs, which are expectorated or passed in the stool, completes the life cycle from humans to freshwater snail to edible fish.

Eosinophilia and lung symptoms mimic TPE, which is due to an allergic response to filaria (*W. bancrofti* or *B. malayi*). TB is unlikely given the history, a negative TT, and lack of typical CXR appearance. Melioidosis comes on acutely and may present with cutaneous as well as pulmonary lesions. On CXR the apices are usually spared.

37. A. Cysticercosis is common in tropical countries and constitutes a major public health problem in Ecuador. It is contracted by ingesting ova of *Taenia solium* from water or food contaminated by infected faeces. Ova can also be ingested by autoinfection (anus to mouth) or by transfer from the unclean hands of others.

After developing in the intestine liberated larvae penetrate the mucosa and lodge mainly in the brain, skin, and subcutaneous tissue. The larvae (*Cysticercus cellulosae*) ultimately become encysted in fibrous tissue masses that eventually calcify. These can often be felt as palpable nodules under the skin or in muscle. When they occur in the brain (neurocysticercosis) they form space-occupying lesions that can cause neurologic signs and symptoms mimicking epilepsy, CVA, brain tumour, tuberculoma, or even chronic brucellosis. The history and the presence of subcutaneous nodules point to the diagnosis in this case. Anti-cysticercal antibodies may be found in blood or CSF while ova of *T. solium* may be found in the stool.

T. saginata (beef tapeworm) does not cause cysticercosis. Distinguish between cysticercosis and taeniasis, each of which represents a different stage in the life cycle of *T. solium*. Cysticercosis is acquired by ingesting the ova of *T.solium*, taeniasis is acquired by ingesting the cysts of *T. solium* or *T. saginta*, which are found in the meat of an intermediate host (pig or cow).

In cysticercosis ingested eggs of *T. solium* ultimately form larval cysts in human tissues, in taeniasis the adult *T. solium* or *T. saginata* lives in the human intestine. Both forms sometimes exist in the same individual.

38. C. Cysticercosis, especially neurocysticercosis, may be treated with PZQ, albendazole, steroids, and surgery. Steroids suppress damaging allergic side effects. Excision of the cyst(s) may also be needed.

Anyone suffering from taeniasis (*T. solium*, *T. saginata*) should be dewormed with PZQ (5–10 mg/kg) or niclosamide (2 g stat) after a light meal. Cimetidine, in contrast to steroids, increases plasma PZQ and albendazole.

39. A. He may have any of the options but is most likely to have *Cyclospora cayetanensis*. This infection of the small bowel must be considered in such a patient even if other parasites are found in the stool. Cryptosporidium may coexist with *C. cayetanensis* in such patients. Usually HIV-AIDS travellers are on co-trimoxazole as a prophylactic against *P. jirovecii*, in which case they are then unlikely to get *C. cayetanensis*. The course of both infections is normally self-limiting in immunocompetent persons.

P. jirovecii is actually a fungus and not a protozoan, but it does not respond to antifungal treatment. It is present in normal lungs and acts as an opportunistic predator in HIV patients, where it often causes pneumocystis pneumonia. It was formerly misnamed *P. carinii*, a protozoan that infects animals.

40. C. Despite denying sexual contact, gonorrhoea is the obvious diagnosis given the incubation period and the symptoms and signs. Appropriate urethral, throat, and rectal swabs should be taken. Gonorrhoeal infection should be treated with appropriate antibiotics.

Chlamydial infection from oral, anal, or vaginal sex is now extremely common and must also be considered. Symptoms appear within 2–6 weeks and not in 2–7 days as with gonorrhea. However, three-quarters of infected women and about half of infected men have no symptoms so the diagnosis of chlamydia is often bacteriological only. Azithromycin or doxycycline twice daily for a week is a sensible treatment.

Lymphogranuloma venereum is a sexually transmitted disease caused by invasive serovars of *Chlamydia trachomatis*. It is endemic in the tropics and usually presents as a small pimple or painless ulcer on the penis (or vagina) that can progress to an inguinal syndrome, between 1 week and 6 months later, with painful adenopathy, systemic illness, and malaise.

Although one swim in the Mekong can cause schistosomiasis (*S. mekongi*) the symptoms and time scale are totally different. HIV does not present like this. This man may also have herpes simplex (HSV-1,HSV-2). This can reactivate in times of stress and should be treated with local antiseptics and acyclovir. Chancroid (*H. ducreyi*) is also a possibility but usually appears as a single small genital lump that rapidly ulcerates. Dysuria is not typical.

41. B. It is important to screen for hepatitis, syphilis, and HIV after the acute infection has been cleared up and repeat the screen 2 months later. Give the patient his test results and warn him to avoid sexual contact with anyone until he is better. It is unethical to inform his wife/partner without discussing it with the patient and getting his consent unless you are certain he will be sexually irresponsible. It is unrealistic to try and trace contacts in this case. Counselling may have little to offer.

42. C. Bites on exposed arms are encountered by >75% of all travellers and it is difficult to avoid scratching them. The time of appearance, the area of travel, and the specific activities of the traveller may suggest other diagnoses. A typical eschar is black in colour.

43. A. *Strongyloides stercoralis* is an intestinal hookworm that often accompanies and is very similar to better known hookworms such as *Ankylostoma duodenale* and *Necator americanus*. It differs from these in that autoinfection can occur. When the parasite is in the infective (filariform) state it can penetrate inwards through the perianal skin after defecation. Autoinfection also occurs in the small intestine when rhabditiform larvae evolve into the filariform type and directly penetrate the mucosa. Eosinophilia can exceed 25,000/mm³ in some cases. Strongyloidosis hyperinfection is a very serious illness (see chapter 4).

44. C. Strongyloides is often characterized by pulmonary symptoms. Sometimes it presents with a transient pruritic intradermal migration of filariform larvae (larva currens) which typically occurs in a white person who resided in South-East Asia many years previously. This was not present in this case. Patients with altered cell-mediated immunity, for example those on steroids or with HIV, are at special risk of hyperinfection if they contract strongyloides. Imported strongyloidosis has a high impact on public health and the mortality rate among patients hospitalized for this condition can be up to 16.7%. Ivermectin 200 µg/kg for 2 days is the treatment of choice.

Amoebiasis is likely to present with chronic diarrhoea or an enlarged tender liver whereas opisthorchiasis (Oriental liver fluke) takes far longer than 3 months to cause symptoms. Giardiasis must also be considered in this case, but it does not account for the presence of pulmonary symptoms.

45. D. Tests for antigens to *S. stercoralis* are about 90% sensitive but not very specific because of cross-reactions with filarial and echinococcal antigens. Nonetheless, when taken in conjunction with a history of travel to endemic areas, ELISA testing is very reliable. An eosinophilia >450 cells/μl is about 38% sensitive and 90% specific for invasive parasitic diseases but does not differentiate between them. Stool examination by concentration methods can show larvae but it may take up to seven or more stool samples to get a positive result. Larvae of *S. stercoralis* may be seen in some cases creeping out of a stool mass in response to the heat of a light bulb (Batemann technique). The D-xylose absorption test may be positive in chronic stronglyoides but it is also positive in many other malabsorption syndromes.

46. B. Neither malaria nor dengue fever occur in Portugal. In view of the number of mosquito bites West Nile fever is most likely. Meningitis, influenza, and other infections may also be considered.

47. C. Specific IgM levels are raised long before IgG. Ideally viral culture of blood, urine, or CSF confirms the diagnosis beyond doubt, but this is slow and not always feasible. A high index of suspicion is based on history, symptoms, and an incubation period of 7–14 days (possibly longer in some cases).

48. B. The symptoms of onchocerciasis take 15–18 months to appear. At this stage there is an allergic reaction to dying and dead microfilariae, with widespread itching and/or redness and itching of the eyes. The condition is confined to West Africa with patchy distribution in parts of central Africa and Yemen (where it is called Sowda).

49. D. Microfilariae may appear in the skin as early as 10–15 months after infection. Adult female worms live for 9–14 years, during which time they release 700–1500 microfilariae per day. Compare this to the prolific 100,000 daily output of *W. bancrofti* (lymphatic filariasis). Onchocercomata (nodules) contain one or two male (3–5cm long) and two or three female (30–80 cm long) worms and may be palpable as fibrous lumps under the skin, especially in regions of the trochanters.

50. C. Even if the patient is HIV negative it is safest to assume she is incubating HIV and has not converted yet. Start post-exposure prophylaxis (PEP) if possible within 2–4 hours. Then bring her home so that she can have adequate access to HAART, get baseline blood tests done, and have a HIV test at 6 weeks, 3 months, and 6 months. Normally one would continue PEP for 1 month. Most infectious disease clinics have protocols tailored to low, high, and moderate risk cases after needlestick injuries. The risk of HIV is very high in sub-Saharan Africa, where many doctors and nurses as well as patients are HIV+. It should be emphasized that the transmission rate of HIV via needlestick injury is very low.

It is important to support the student and her family as much as possible (personal case).

51. B. Chagas' disease was considered the most likely. Achalasia, hysteria, and cancer were also considered in that order. She made a good recovery after a Ramstedt-type operation.

Chagas' disease is prevalent in South America. It is acquired by rubbing trypomastigote laden faeces of *T. cruzi* into a break in the skin or into a mucus membrane, often the conjunctiva. It is also acquired by drinking sugar cane or fruit juice contaminated with triatomid bugs, as a congenital infection, and more and more in any country by blood transfusion.

Trypomastigotes develop in the host into amistogotes, which invade muscle and neuroglia, causing problems later such as atrial fibrillation, mega-oesophagus, mega-colon, or even mega-ureter. The walls and ceilings of adobes in South America may contain thousands of the bugs, resulting in a blood loss in local people in excess of 2 ml per night.

Chagas' disease is an increasing problem, particularly in the USA and the Iberian peninsula, where there is an influx of immigrants from Latin America (personal case).

52. A. Candida is the most likely diagnosis and should be treated with nystatin. Salt water mouthwashes and triamcinolone lozenges may also help. Herpes causes circumoral ulcers but does not cause white plaques or swallowing difficulties.

Leukoplakia plaques do not scrape off easily. A sore mouth, plus red or purple lumps on the tongue or roof of the mouth, suggest Kaposi sarcoma. Red plaques are also seen in candidiasis.

53. B. Fungal infections are rare in travellers and usually affect either the lungs or skin. Fusarosis has come to prominence not only because is it likely to appear in the immunocompromised but also because it can manifest itself in normal people, especially in those who wear contact lenses, as an iritis, corneal ulceration, and eye pain. Consequent infectious keratitis can result in permanent loss of vision. Fusarosis should be suspected in anyone who has contact with soil or sand and in whom topical antibiotics fail to clear up 'conjunctivitis'. Topical and systemic antifungal agents are indicated. Infected contact lens fluid is also an important cause of the condition.

PSYCHIATRIC AND BEHAVIOURAL PROBLEMS

1. **The Jerusalem syndrome is an acute psychotic syndrome brought on by**
   A. Taking illicit drugs
   B. A reaction to antimalarials, especially mefloquine
   C. A misplaced desire to die for a political/religious cause
   D. An identifcation of self with messianic or biblical incidents

2. **Air rage is most common**
   A. On long-haul flights
   B. As an alcohol-related incident
   C. In a person with a psychiatric history
   D. In someone who has had an incident of air rage previously

3. **Apart from alcohol the most common cause of air rage is**
   A. Smoking or the desire to smoke
   B. Fear of missing connecting flights
   C. Fear of missing appointments at destination
   D. Misuse of medication such as antidepressants drugs

4. **What is the most common psychiatric reason for the medical evacuation of travellers?**
   A. Substance abuse
   B. Adjustment disorder
   C. Acute psychotic episode
   D. Reaction to antimalarials, e.g. mefloquine

5. **The most common causes of confusion in non-evacuees returning from the tropics are**
   A. Culture shock, anxiety, maladjustment
   B. Licit drugs taken while overseas, e.g. acetohexamide, antimalarials, alcohol
   C. Illicit drugs taken while in the tropics
   D. Infectious conditions, e.g. typhoid

6. **Which of the following is the most common psychiatric disorder in young travellers (20–30 years old) who have just returned from a holiday in Asia or Africa?**
   A. Anxiety
   B. Depression
   C. Acute psychosis
   D. Distressing flash-backs

7. **Post-traumatic stress (PTS) disorder is typically characterized by**
   A. Outbursts of unprovoked anger
   B. Depression
   C. Insomnia, nightmares, flashbacks
   D. Bouts of trembling/fatigue/dyspnoea

8. **Which of the following is the most common finding in expatriates with chronic fatigue syndrome (CFS)?**
   A. Fatigue
   B. Insomnia
   C. Vague pains and aches
   D. Muscle weakness

9. **The most common psychological problem faced by expatriates working in a crisis situation for 6–12 months is**
   A. Interpersonal strife with other expatriates
   B. Loneliness
   C. Depression
   D. Fear for personal security

10. **The most frequently encountered form of distress during commercial air travel for which a nurse or doctor is called is**
    A. Impatience/aggression
    B. Hyperventilation
    C. Pseudocardiac pain
    D. Repeated demands for attention

11. **The fear of flying**
    A. Affects over 50% of travellers
    B. Seldom coexists with other phobias
    C. Is seldom alleviated by psychological means alone
    D. Is generally centered on several issues, such as crashing, lack of control, confinement, questioning the pilot's ability

12. Neuropsychiatric problems (NPPs) in travellers

    A. Are less common than in the general non-travelling public

    B. Account for the majority of medical problems seen in international airports

    C. Are frequently due to taking illicit drugs

    D. Constitute a small minority of medical evacuations for expatriates

13. Which is the most significant cause of psychosocial problems in seafarers?

    A. Adapting to new crew members

    B. Accepting inequalities in pay

    C. Long absences from home

    D. Attitude of senior officers

1. D. In some people a visit to Jerusalem engenders such deep religious emotions as to make them acutely delusional. They identify themselves with the prophets of old, dress in flowing robes, and act as if they were present in messianic times. Some may have pre-existing psychiatric problems, others appear as normal pilgrims, still others travel to Jerusalem without any religious pre-conceptions. A similar overwhelming response to Renaissance art has been seen in tourists visiting Florence, the so-called Florence or Stendhal syndrome. Stendhal wrote movingly of the beauties of Florence. Many over-the-top 'art lovers' have latent psychiatric problems.

2. B. Excessive intake of alcohol before and/or during the flight is by far the most common precipitating factor for air rage. Despite the absence of objective evidence it is said of alcohol that 'two on the ground equals one in the air'.

3. A. Smoking or the desire to smoke comprised 40% of the total number of air rage cases in one survey (260 incidents). Smoking may also endanger the whole flight if matches or cigarettes are disposed of carelessly in the toilet.

4. A. In one series of evacuations substance abuse accounted for almost 30% of the cases and there is no reason to suspect that this is still not so. Note that mefloquine causes neuropsychiatric effects in one person per 200–250 (therapeutic dose) and one person per 10,000 (prophylactic dose). Neuropsychiatric problems account for 15–20% of medical evacuations (chapter 13).

5. B. Adverse reactions to prescribed drugs, e.g. antimalarials, or an inadvertant overdose are important causes of post-travel problems. Mistaking acetohexamide for acetazolamide can cause hypoglycaemia and over-indulgence in alcohol alone or in combination or other drugs may also result in the 'confused traveller'. Illicit drug taking is second in this category of traveller. Typhoid encephalopathy has also been reported in returned travellers.

6. A. Anxiety was the major problem found in a series of returned young travellers who presented to a psychiatric clinic in Israel. The male:female ratio as was 2:1. Almost all returnees had visited India or South-East Asia and almost one-third had taken illicit drugs varying from cannabis to hashish to LSD. A small number presented with acute psychosis. The contribution of mefloquine to the behavioural changes was uncertain in these patients.

7. C. Post-traumatic stress is becoming more frequent in travellers especially in humanitarian aid workers, in those who report on natural and man-made disasters, and in military personnel. The initiating incident(s)—often borne with apparent fortitude—is pushed into the subconscious. Typically the sufferer is reluctant to talk about what happened but panic attacks, anxiety, a broken sleep pattern, and distorted dreams and nightmares can start anytime, even years afterwards. Flashbacks may be triggered by things that remind the patient of the original experience. Counselling, psychotherapy, and encouraging the patient to repeat the story will all help. Psychotropic drugs are contraindicated. Any of the other options may also occur.

8. C. CFS is very common in expatriates. Symptoms are varied and often vague. Mostly they complain of a wide variety of somatoform symptoms, e.g. pains and aches, and chronic diarrhoea. Symptoms may even mimic an acute abdomen. Fatigue is sometimes present but not always prominent.

Frequently expatriates with CFS are diligent and conscientious workers. The chief thing to do is to exclude organic disease (amoebiasis, anaemia, neurocysticercosis). It is said that 90% of expatriates with CFS have something to gain from the illness. It is well known that working overseas is a ploy used by many to escape personal difficulties at home, but they soon find out that they have merely changed the sky overhead (Ovid).

9. A. Although loneliness, anger, anxiety and depression can all occur, the most common problem one faces is personality clashes with co-workers, especially with other expatriate workers (personal review of returned aid workers, unpublished).

10. B. Episodes of overbreathing are often triggered by an accumulation of stressors before and during the flight, e.g. long queues at check-in, delayed departure, last-minute rushing, arguments about overweight luggage, poor seating arrangements in the aeroplane, and the indifference of flight attendants. The other options occur less frequently.

11. D. Generally fears are multifactorial. Fear of flying affects 10–40% of people and as many as 46% of these will have experienced other phobias, e.g. agoraphobia or claustrophobia. Psychological treatment has a high success rate.

12. C. Illicit drug taking was found in 22% of a cohort of 2500 young (mostly 20–25 years old) travellers who took part in a postal survey conducted by doctors at the Bnai Zion Medical Center, Israel. This study showed that 11.3% suffered from NPPs which is far higher than in the general population. NPPs are characterized by many symptoms varying from depression, anxiety, insomnia, and dizziness to manifest psychosis. Most medical problems at international airports apart from myocardial infarction are trivial. Only 1.1% of 3350 people who sought medical assistance in Bahrain International Airport in 2005 presented as an NPP. It should be remembered that travel may merely unmask an underlying NPP so that an absolute link between travel and NPP cannot be asserted unequivocally.

13. A. Adapting to new crew members is an important stressor as it is in any team, whether on land or sea. Other stressors include age, race, pay discrimination, long hours, the lack of sick leave, confrontations with suprvisors and/or passengers, and the uncertainty of the length of each trip. Adapting to life on shore is also an important stressor. Medical care is only one element of the overall management, which involves employers, senior staff, trade unions, welfare agencies, and even consultation with other crew members.

DRUGS AND TRAVEL

Travel medicine is unique in that drugs and vaccines are given to perfectly healthy people either to prevent an illness that they have only a remote chance of acquiring, e.g. Japanese encephalitis, or to treat an illness that they do not already have, e.g. travellers' diarrhoea. It is therefore incumbent on travel health advisors to be fully familiar with the nature of the drugs/vaccines they use, the indications and contraindications and the individual cost/benefit ratios.

It is useful to give travellers a printout about any drugs prescribed so that they can refer to it when overseas, where medical help may not be always available. It is also useful to know the cost of medicines because this may play a part in choosing a generic versus a proprietary brand. In the opinion of many, buying drugs on the internet is not to be encouraged because of doubts about quality and effectiveness.

Purchasing drugs abroad may be easy but beware of the profusion of illicit and counterfeit drugs which are for sale at deceptively cheap prices. There are electronic methods being developed so that any drug purchased anywhere has an identifiable secure ID. However, such methods are not available in the places where they are most needed.

Some drugs deteriorate over time, especially in warm climates, so that if the patient is given a large supply before travel, e.g doxycycline, there may be difficulty in storing it correctly.

Finally, carriage of drugs across borders is fraught with danger, even if the drugs are accompanied by a doctor's letter. All medications, including codeine, should be declared at Customs if problems are to be avoided.

Antimalarials

1. **Chloroquine-resistant falciparum malaria (CRFM) occurs in**
   A. Haiti
   B. Egypt
   C. Vietnam
   D. Yemen

2. **What is the approximate incidence of serious adverse effects when taking chloroquine to prevent malaria?**
   A. 1 per 100
   B. 1 per 500
   C. 1 per 5000
   D. 1 per 10,000

3. **What is the approximate incidence of serious adverse effects when taking mefloquine to prevent malaria?**
   A. 1 per 100
   B. 1 per 500
   C. 1 per 5000
   D. 1 per 10,000

4. **Doxycycline is regarded as an excellent antimalarial prophylactic because**
   A. It gives excellent protection against all forms of malaria
   B. It gives excellent protection against CRFM
   C. It has a half-life of 48 hours
   D. It is active against malarial hypnozoites (dormant forms in the liver)

5. **Doxycycline 100 mg daily**
   A. Is an effective prophylaxis against rickettsial infection
   B. Reduces the transmission rate of the HIV virus
   C. Causes fewer adverse reactions than either chloroquine or proguanil
   D. Is safe throughout pregnancy

6. **Which of the following interact with doxycycline?**
   A. Anticonvulsants, e.g. phenytoin, carbamazepine
   B. Anticoagulants, e.g. warfarin
   C. Antifungal agents, e.g. nystatin
   D. Depot oestrogens

7. **Doxycycline is used alone to treat**
   A. Malaria
   B. Lyme disease
   C. Brucellosis
   D. Gonorrhoea

8. **Which of the following should you tell your patients about doxycycline?**
   A. It is best to take doxycycline just before retiring at night
   B. It is important to take doxycycline with food
   C. Prolonged courses may exacerbate bronchial asthma
   D. It causes photosensitivity in about 20% of recipients

9. **Dermatological problems occur most frequently after**
   A. Doxycycline
   B. Mefloquine
   C. Chloroquine
   D. Atovaquone/proguanil

10. **When doxycycline is used as a malarial prophylactic it**
    A. May facilitate vaginal herpes in some women
    B. May aggravate existing endometriosis
    C. May facilitate vaginal candidiasis
    D. Has a proved long-term (6–12 months) safety profile

11. **Atovaquone 250 mg/proguanil 100 mg (AP, Malarone™) appears to provide the best protection against**
    A. *P. falciparum*
    B. *P. vivax*
    C. *P. ovale*
    D. *P. malaria*

12. **Atovaquone 250 mg/proguanil 100 mg (Malarone™) is contraindicated in**
    A. The elderly (>65 years)
    B. Children (<12 years)
    C. Those who weigh < 50 kg
    D. Those with mild renal impairment

13. **Which of the following is true of atovaquone 250 mg/proguanil 100 mg (Malarone™)?**
    A. Resistance by *P. falciparum* has been authentically reported
    B. Atovaquone is mainly metabolized in the liver
    C. Absorption is independent of food
    D. Atovaquone 250 mg/proguanil 100 mg (Malarone™) the first line treatment of toxoplasmosis

14. **Atovaquone 250 mg/proguanil 100 mg (Malarone™)**
    A. Causes adverse effects more often in males than in females
    B. May cause methaemoglobinaemia with prolonged use (>4 weeks)
    C. Induces electrophysiologicial asymptomatic cardiac conduction defects in >40% of users
    D. Interacts with warfarin

15. **Which of the following is true of malaria prophylaxis?**
    A. Appropriate chemoprophylaxis is by far the best way of avoiding malaria
    B. Adverse effects are almost twice as common when using a recognized current chemoprophylactic agent as when using a placebo
    C. Gastrointestinal symptoms vary widely between chemoprophylactics, e.g. between doxycycline and mefloquine
    D. Malarone™ (AP, atovaquone/proguanil) is active both at the liver (causal) and asexual blood stage of *P. falciparum*

16. **Match the mode of action with commonly used malarial prophylactics**

    A. Chloroquine   1. Competes with the parasite binding to haeme
    B. Proguanil   2. Interferes with parasite ribosomes
    C. Mefloquine   3. Interferes with degradation of haemoglobin
    D. Doxycycline   4. Interferes with folate metabolism

17. **Proguanil (Paludrine™) prophylaxis should be started**

    A. 4 weeks before entering a malarious area
    B. 2 weeks before entering a malarious area
    C. 2 days before entering a malarious area
    D. On entering a malarious area

18. **Proguanil (Paludrine™)**

    A. Is contraindicated in pregnancy
    B. Is a used widely to treat mild malaria
    C. Prevents relapsing malaria
    D. Is a causal prophylactic

19. **Prominent side effects of proguanil include**

    A. Photosensitization
    B. Mouth ulcers
    C. Excessive hair growth
    D. Loss of libido (long term)

20. **Which of the following has a half-life of about 3 weeks?**

    A. Mefloquine
    B. Doxycycline
    C. Atovaquone/proguanil
    D. Chloroquine

21. **Which of the following is true of primaquine?**

    A. Primaquine is effective against erythrocytic forms of all types of malaria
    B. Primaquine is highly effective against the gametocyte phase of most plasmodia
    C. Primaquine reaches peak plasma levels 24 hours after oral ingestion
    D. Primaquine should be given parenterally in severe malaria

22. **Those most likely to have glucose 6-phosphate dehydrogenase (G6PD) deficiency are**

    A. Long-term travellers to tropical countries
    B. Expatriates living in the Mediterranean littoral
    C. Visitors to blood relatives in the Middle East
    D. Travellers known to be sensitive to sulphonamides

23. **Haemolysis with primaquine in G6PD-deficient people**
    A. Is more common in females than in males
    B. Is independent of the drug dosage
    C. Is greater in reticulocytes than in older red cells
    D. Is greater in affected whites than in affected blacks

24. **If you had to use one of the following as a malarial chemoprophylactic which would you choose for an adult going to Assam?**
    A. Quinine
    B. Artemisinins
    C. Azithromycin
    D. Amodiaquine

25. **Eradication of *P. vivax* infection is best accomplished using**
    A. Chloroquine for at least 1 month
    B. Chloroquin and proguanil for at least 1 month
    C. No drugs until and unless clinical malaria
    D. Primaquine alone or in combination with chloroquine

26. **Which of these regimes is your preferred SBET for malaria anywhere in the world?**
    A. Mefloquine (Lariam™): 100 mg/kg in split doses 6 hours apart
    B. Chloroquine 900 mg base stat
    C. ACT
    D. Atovaquone-proguanil (Malarone™): 4 tablets daily × 7 days

27. **The preferred SBET for malaria in all stages of pregnancy is**
    A. Artemisinins
    B. Chloroquine
    C. Quinine
    D. Azithromycin

28. **Travellers who are allergic to sulpha drugs should not take**
    A. Malarone
    B. Maloprim
    C. Fansidar
    D. Euratesim™ or Riamet™

29. **In comparing Eurartesim™, Coartem™ and Riamet™**
    A. Any of these can be used in SBET for *P. falciparum*
    B. All three are best taken with a fatty meal or drink
    C. All three are roughly equally effective against re-infection
    D. Only Eurartesim is recommended against *P. vivax*

30. Coarscum™ (amodiaquine hydrochloride 270 mg; artesunate 100 mg)

A. Is closely related to chloroquine

B. Is more effective than other ACTs in clearing *P. falciparum*

C. Is less stable than dihydroartemisin

D. Significantly decreases bioavailability when there are fatty foods in the intestine

31. Artemisinins

A. Cause an accumulation of haeme in malarial parasites

B. Are folic acid inhibitors

C. Are derived from the bark of the cinchona tree

D. Are only available in parenteral form

32. When treating uncomplicated *P. falciparum* malaria

A. Artemisinins alone give the best results

B. Quinine alone gives the best results

C. Piperaquine (PQP) is a safe replacement for artemisinins

D. ACT is the preferred option

33. Which of the following chemoprophylactics is the most appropriate for someone going to Afghanistan?

A. Proguanil and chloroquin

B. Atovaquone plus proguanil

C. Mefloquine

D. No antimalarial necessary

Drugs in travellers' diarrhoea

1. Quinolone resistance is becoming an important consideration in treating diarrhoea due to

A. *Isospora belli*

B. *Cyclospora cayetanensis*

C. *Cryptosporidium parvum*

D. *Campylobacter jejuni*

2. Match the disease with the treatment. Treatment options may be used once, more than once, or not at all

A. Amoebic dysentery   1. Praziquantel

B. Schistosomiasis   2. Ivermectin

C. Typhoid   3. Ceftriaxone

D. Filariasis   4. Metronidazole

3. **An adult traveller has severe bloody diarrhoea while travelling in a remote area. He has a well-stocked medical bag. He should treat himself with**

   A. ORS only

   B. ORS plus a fluoroquinolone

   C. ORS plus loperamide (Imodium)

   D. ORS plus a fluoroquinolone plus azithromycin

4. **Trimethoprim-sulfamethoxazole (co-trimoxazole,TMP-SMX, Septrin®) is an excellent treatment for diarrhoea due to**

   A. Recurrent amoebiasis

   B. *Cryptosporidium parvum*

   C. *Non-cholera vibrio*

   D. *Cyclospora cayetanensis*

5. **Loperamide (Imodium™) in TD**

   A. Is both an intestinal antimotility and antisecretory agent

   B. Is safe in reduced doses for children <2 years of age

   C. Is less effective in treating diarrhoea than diphenyoxylate/atropine (Lomotil™)

   D. Potentiates the depressant effects of alcohol

6. **Which of the following can cause a black tongue, blackened stools, and tinnitus?**

   A. Bismuth subsalicylate (BSS, Pepto-Bismol™)

   B. Imodium™

   C. Acetyl salicylic acid

   D. Quinine

7. **BSS should not be taken with**

   A. Proton pump inhibitors

   B. Antidepressants

   C. Alcohol

   D. Aspirin

8. **Which is the most important in preventing TD?**

   A. An antimotility drug

   B. Good personal hygiene

   C. Eating only in clean places

   D. Eating only well-cooked food

9. **Chemoprophylaxis against TD**
   A. Is recommended for anyone going to a high-risk area >4 weeks
   B. Should never be recommended
   C. Creates the risk of promoting drug resistance
   D. With prebiotics is considered a good alternative to synthetic medicines

10. **Which is your drug of choice in non-bloody TD?**
    A. Co-trimoxazole
    B. Kaolin
    C. Loperamide
    D. Diphenoxylate with atropine (Lomotil™)

11. **Which is the best in the prevention/amelioration of TD?**
    A. Transcutaneous patch vaccines
    B. *Lactobacillus acidophilus*
    C. *Saccharomyces boulardii*
    D. Tap water

12. **Which of the following is true of Rifaximin?**
    A. Rifaximin well absorbed orally
    B. Rifaximin has a high potential for inducing cross-resistance to rifampicin and rifamycin
    C. Rifaximin is useful in dysentery
    D. Rifaximin can be taken with or without food

13. **Rifaximin**
    A. Interferes with oral contraceptives
    B. Is permitted in children over 1 year
    C. Is generally effective in TD caused by quinolone resistant Campylobacter
    D. Has been approved and used in Italy for over 20 years

14. **Rifaximin has been shown to be most effective against**
    A. *Giardia lamblia*
    B. *Isospora belli*
    C. ETEC
    D. Cryptosporidia

15. **When rifaximin is used as a preventative against TD**
    A. Give it daily for 1 week prior to entering a highly endemic area for moderate prophylaxis
    B. Give 500 mg 24 hours before probable exposure to provide good prophylaxis
    C. Give >500 mg daily for 2 weeks starting 3 days before departure for excellemt prophlylaxis
    D. Results are no better than with a placebo

Miscellaneous

1. **Trimethoprim-sulfamethoxazole (TMP-SMX, co-trimoxazole) is useful in treating**
   A. *Mycoplasma pneumoniae*
   B. *Shigella*
   C. *S. typhi*
   D. Myiasis

2. **Erythromycin is very useful in treating**
   A. Legionnaire's disease *(Legionella pneumophila)*
   B. Shigella
   C. *S. typhi*
   D. Myiasis

3. **Erythromycin is a preferred antibiotic in the treatment of**
   A. Pontiac fever
   B. *Mycoplasma pneumoniae*
   C. *P. jirovecii* pneumonia
   D. Leptospirosis

4. **Match each condition with a drug that is useful in its treatment. Drug options may be used once, more than once, or not at all**
   A. Schistosomiasis   1. Mefloquine
   B. Filariasis   2. Artemisinins
   C. Malaria   3. TMP-SMX
   D. *Campylobacter jejuni*   4. Doxycycline

5. **The best drug to treat schistosomiasis is**
   A. PZQ (Distocide™)
   B. Ivermectin (Mectizan™)
   C. Artemisinins/lumefantrine or piperaquine (Coartem™, Riamet™, Eurartesim™)
   D. Doxycycline (Vibramycin™, Bymycin™)

6. **Which of the following is true of drugs in schistosomiasis?**
   A. PZQ kills all stages of the schistosomule
   B. Artemisinin derivatives kill only mature schistosomules
   C. Mefloquine and artemisinin derivatives can substantially reduce the worm burden
   D. Corticosteroids can precipitate a Mazotti-type reaction in cases of schistosomiasis

7. Ivermectin is used to treat

A. *Schistosoma japonicum*
B. Taeniasis
C. Loa loa (African eye worm)
D. Combined loa loa and onchocerciasis (both filarial infestations)

8. Ivermectin is effective in treating

A. Scabies
B. Ascariasis
C. Amoebiasis
D. Cryptosporidium

9. Which is the most useful of these for the immediate treatment of HAPE?

A. Acetazolamide
B. Ginkgo biloba
C. Dexamethasone
D. Nifedipine

10. Photosensitivity

A. Only affects areas exposed to light
B. Implies a priming agent, e.g. a drug
C. Is quicker to occur in older people
D. Only occurs in fair-skinned people

11. Which of the following is most likely to cause photosensitivity?

A. Tetracycline
B. Chloroquine
C. Mefloquine
D. Acetazolamide

12. Miltefosine is used in the

A. Treatment of CL and VL
B. Treatment of MDRTB
C. Prophylaxis of malaria
D. Prophylaxis of TD

DRUGS AND TRAVEL

Antimalarials

1. C. Vietnam and the borders of Thailand are areas where resistance to antimalarials often begins. CRFM is widespread apart from parts of the Arabian peninsula and central America. Resistance is linked to amino acid substitutions in specific encoding genes of the parasite.

2. D. 1 per 10,000 travellers on chloroquin is hospitalized for serious adverse physical or psychological side effects.

3. D. This is the same as for chloroquin. Chemoprophylaxis can sometimes do more harm than good and thus should be individually tailored to the traveller's destination, activities, length of stay, and past history.

4. B. Protection against CRFM is the major advantage of doxycycline. Its main mode of action is on the parasite ribosome in the blood phase. Although doxycycline is almost as effective against *P. vivax* as against *P. falciparum* in the blood phase, it fails to affect hypnozoites and so does not prevent recurrent malaria. The half-life of doxycycline is 18–22 hours and this ensures once-daily dosage. There is no such thing as a 100% effective antimalarial chemoprophylactic. However, if the correct one is taken in accordance with the manufacturer's instructions the risk of malaria may be reduced 10-fold. Thus when the estimated risk of getting malaria in a specific area is 1 in 10,000, the risk may reduced to 1:100,000.

5. A. Doxycycline is an effective prophylactic against rickettsia, relapsing fever, and cholera, and perhaps against some bacterial diarrhoeas. It is also used >6 months in acne and Q-fever endocarditis. There is no evidence that it affects HIV transmission. It is not used in pregnancy because of its effects on foetal bone development, a judgment contested by Lars Rombo (Sweden). Adverse reactions are more frequent than with other prophylactic drugs.

6. A. Anticonvulsants, including barbiturates, induce enzymatic destruction of doxycycline in the liver and therefore the dosage of doxycycline may need to be increased. The usual dose of doxycycline is 2 mg base/kg body weight per day up to 100 mg.

7. B. Doxycycline 100 mg bid for 10–30 days gives excellent results in early Lyme disease. It is used in conjunction with quinine in treating malaria and with streptomycin, rifampicin, or gentamycin in brucellosis. It is used with ceftriaxone in the treatment of gonorrhea.

Doxycycline is used also in the treatment of a variety of tick- and louse-borne diseases as well as in treating entities such as chlamydia, syphilis, and acne. Doxycycline is probably the best choice if you could only bring one drug with you when travelling extensively in the tropics.

8. B. Nausea is by far the most common adverse side effect of doxycycline and this is dramatically reduced by taking the drug with food. In the prevention of malaria it should be taken at roughly the same time each day and never within 30 minutes of lying down for fear of reflux oesophagitis. Photosensitivity probably occurs in up to 3.0% of users. A sunblock (SPF > 20) should be used when exposed to sunlight. Warn those going on sun or mountain climbing holidays.

9. A. Photosensitivity is a possibility when taking doxycycline as a malarial prophylactic in the recommended adult dose of 100 mg daily. One study showed that dermatological problems with doxycycline were significantly greater than with any other antimalarial drug (12.5% as against 1.5%).

10. C. Like many antibiotics doxycycline facilitates the development of vaginal candidiasis but has no link to herpes. Doxycycline, along with other antibiotics such as amoxycillin and erythromycin, alters gut flora and may interfere with the absorption of oestrogen. Although this is most unlikely to interfere with the efficacy of an oestrogen-containing OC yet, should a pregnancy occur, the prescriber may face unpleasant legal consequences. However, in March 2011, when commenting on drug interactions with hormonal contraception, the Royal College of Obstetricians and Gynaecologists stated that 'women on non-enzyme-inducing antibiotics are no longer required to take additional precautions during or after the course'. Nonetheless, in the current litigious climate some still advise abstinence or the use of an alternative contraceptive for the first 3 weeks of doxycycline usage. Doxycycline has no effect on endometriosis. Long-term safety >6 months has not been definitively established and the long-term use of some tetracycline derivatives, e.g. minocycline, has been shown to be associated with serious adverse effects such as autoimmune hepatitis and lupus. Non-compliance with the daily dose of doxycycline has been found to be the main reason for failure of doxycycline to protect against malaria.

11. A. AP has a protective efficacy of about 96% against *P. falciparum* but only 84% against *P. vivax*. There are no firm figures available for its efficacy against *P. ovale*, *P. malariae*, or *P. knowlesi*. AP is a causal prophylactic, that is, it is effective against the tissue stages of the four major malaria-causing plasmodia. At the liver stage it appears to be more effective against *P. falciparum* than *P. vivax*. Unfortunately it is not significantly effective against the liver-stage hypnozites of *P. vivax* or *P. ovale* and is therefore unable to prevent relapsing malaria.

12. D. AP is contraindicated when the creatinine clearance is <30 ml/min, presumably because cycloguanil (active ingredient of proguanil) is excreted in the urine. Currently AP is not recommended for prophylaxis of malaria in children <3 years or in those who weigh less than 11 kg. Several reports confirm its safety in the healthy elderly and in children (11–40 kg).

13. A. The first case of Malarone™ resistance in a traveller was reported from Lagos, Nigeria. Currently there are many citations of proved treatment resistance. Most, but not all, are related to point mutations at codon 268 of cytochrome b in the parasites' mitochondria. Atovaquone is lipophilic and best taken with food or milk. It is mostly excreted unchanged into the faeces. AP is a second-line treatment for toxoplasmosis. Trimethoprim-sulfamethoxazole (TMP-SMX) is still the first choice. AP (four tablets/day for 3 days, adult dose) is a good treatment for malaria but has been superseded by artemisinins.

14. D. The proguanil component competes with warfarin for carriage by plasma albumin and so may cause bleeding in those on warfarin. Methaemoglobinaemia occurs in up to 13% of those on daily primaquine for up to a year but not in those on Malarone™. More adverse effects occur in females than in males after either AP (Malarone™) or mefloquine (Lariam™). This is especially so if the BMI is <20 kg/m^2. Cardiac conduction abnormalities have been reported after most antimalarials. Prolongation of the QTc interval >500 ms is regarded as unacceptable. The danger here is of sudden adult death syndrome (SADS), typically triggered by excitement, exercise, or even a sudden shock, e.g. unexpected ringing of a phone. This is not a problem with Malarone™ unless the traveller already has a cardiac electrophysiological anomaly.

15. D. Malarone can be used both for prophylaxis and treatment of malaria and is especially efficacious against *P. falciparum*. It is mildly active against liver forms but not against liver hypnozoites and this must be borne in mind in the febrile returned traveller. For example, *P. vivax* malaria may suddenly appear in personnel returning from a tour of duty in Asia although Malarone™ has been taken conscientiously. Contrary to what is commonly held, gastrointestinal problems are not significantly different using different drugs. Schlagenhauf et al. have shown, in a pre-travel group, that adverse effects occurred in 16% of those given a placebo, which rose to a maximum of 24% in those given chloroquine and proguanil. The only 100% method of avoiding malaria is to avoid being bitten by an infective anopheles mosquito.

16. Answers:

A-1. Chloroquine, a 4-aminoquinolone derivative, inhibits haeme polymerase and thus prevents the parasite from converting haeme that is toxic to the parasite into a non-toxic parasite pigment.

B-4. Proguanil (like pyrimethamine) inhibits dihydrofolate reductase in both parasite and host. This leads to a deficiency of tetrahydrofolate, which is needed for normal parasite schizogony. Plasmodia, unlike humans and animals, cannot make use of preformed folate. Folate supplements should be given to those on long-term proguanil.

C-1. Mefloquine probably acts by competing with parasite protein for haeme binding, resulting in a product toxic to the parasite.

D-2. Doxycycline interferes with parasite ribosomal activity in the blood phase.

17. C. Paludrine can be started 48 hours before entering a malarious area, although current practice is to give it several weeks beforehand.

18. D. Proguanil is the safest of all antimalarials. It is a synthetic derivative of pyrimidine and its active ingredient, cycloguanil, has schizontocidal effects on the primary tissue stages of *P. falciparum*, *P. vivax*, and *P. ovale*. It is therefore a causal prophylactic. However, like doxycycline, it does not affect liver hypnozoites and so does not prevent relapsing malaria. It can be given in normal or greater than normal doses to pregnant women and given in reduced doses to children <14 years old. A note of caution: cycloguanil may be reduced to less than 50% of what is expected in late pregnancy and in women on OCs.

In chloroquine-sensitive areas daily proguanil is used together with weekly chloroquine (300 mg base, adult dose) as a malaria chemoprophylactic. Contrary to reports in the 1940s it is not a treatment drug nor, on its own, a satisfactory prophylactic aganst malaria (personal view).

19. B. Mouth ulcers occasionally occur and can be very annoying. Other gastrointestinal upsets, e.g. nausea or heartburn, are usually avoided by taking the progaunil with or after food. Hair loss is sometimes seen, especially in those of Asian origin. Occasionally urticarial reactions can occur. Loss of libido has not been reported.

20. A. The half-lives are as follows: mefloquine 14–24 days, doxycycline 18–22 hours, atovaquone™ 2–3 days, proguanil 17 hours, chloroquine 30–60 days.

21. B. Primaquine is an 8-aminoquinolone that is highly effective against exoerythrocytic forms of *P. falciparum*, *P. vivax*, and *P. knowlesi* malaria and against the hepatic phase of the relapsing malarias (*P. vivax*, *P. ovale*). It is used for 'terminal prophylaxis' against the latter in a dosage of 20–30 mg/day. Clinical malaria caused by *P. vivax* or *P. ovale*, whether a primary attack or relapse, should be treated with a course of 10 mg/kg chloroquin base orally. Primaquine reaches peak plasma levels in 6 hours and is only given orally. Parenteral primaquine can have profound effects on the ECG.

Since it has insignificant activity against the asexual blood forms of the parasite primaquine is always used in conjunction with a blood schizonticide and not as a single agent. Primaquine should not be used in G6PD deficiency for fear of inducing intravascular haemolysis.

22. C. There is a high incidence of G6PD deficiency in Iranians, native Africans and their descendants, Greeks, Sephardic Jews, and Sardinians. Red cells deficient in G6PD are sensitive to 8-aminoquinolones, e.g. primaquine, sulphonamides, PAS, aspirin, acetazolamide, and fava beans. Haemolysis can be very severe in such cases. Note that sensitivity to sulphonamides does not imply coexisting G6PD deficiency.

23. D. Affected whites whose ancestors came from the Mediterranean littoral are more sensitive to haemolysis by primaquine than similarly affected blacks. The reasons are unclear. Males constitute the vast majority of symptomatic cases because of the recessive X-linked pattern of G6PD transmission. The greater the dose the greater the haemolysis but 15 mg daily is well tolerated by many G6PD-deficient people. Old red cells contain less G6PD and are more susceptible to haemolysis. Reticulocytes are relatively resistant.

24. C. Assam has a high incidence of *P. falciparum* so using any of the above is less than ideal. However, azithromycin is the best of those listed since it gives 70–83% protection against *P. falciparum*. Azithromycin gives >90% protection against *P. vivax*, the most common type of malaria in the rest of India .In addition it is safe in pregnancy and in children. Currently artemisinins and other qinghaosu derivatives are only used in the treatment of malaria. Quinine is not used because of its short half-life and amodiaquine, while still used extensively in treating malaria in West Africa, is considered too dangerous for prophylaxis (liver damage, agranulocytosis, lupus erythematosus).

25. D. Primaquine and tafenoquine are the only drugs that can eradicate the hypnozoite stage of *P. vivax*. Either primaquine (15–30 mg/day for 2 weeks) alone or, better still, in combination with chloroquin, can be used as a radical cure in symptomatic persons or as 'terminal prophylaxis' in asymptomatic persons who are leaving an endemic area and want to prevent later relapses. We do not understand why hypnozoites change into merozoites which actually cause the relapse.

26. C. SBET is used when moderate to high fever occurs suddenly at least 7 days after possible exposure to malaria. The traveller should be in a remote malarious location where medical help is not available within 24 hours. SBET implies that the user is well instructed prior to travel. Clearly SBET must be with a different drug to any chemoprophylactic being taken. Suggested regimes in order of preference :

ACT, e.g. Eurartesim™ (dihydroartemisin, DHA/piperaquine PQP 20/160 or 40/160) one tablet daily for 3 consecutive days, Coartem™ or Riamet™ (artemether/lumefantrine 20/120) four tablets with food repeated 6 times over 60 hours),

Malarone™ (250/100), four tablets as a single dose on 3 consecutive days. Lariam™ (15 mg/kg, do not exceed four 250 mg tablets). Remember mefloquine resistance is now spreading beyond the Thai borders.

Not generally recommmended: Fansidar™ (sulfadoxine 500 mg and pyrimethamine 25 mg) six tablets stat quinine 400 mg tid × 3 days plus doxycycline 100 mg bid × 7 days. Quinine 600 mg is given in hospital. A lower dose is used in SBET to limit side effects, especially tinnitus.

27. C. Quinine 600 mg 3 times daily is the preferred option while seeking urgent medical attention (Travax, 2011). Chloroquine alone is only effective in a few places (Arabian peninsula, parts of Central and of South America). Azithromycin is acceptable in pregnancy but is a weak antimalarial. Artimisinins are only recommended in the second half of pregnancy (WHO).

28. C. Fansidar contains sulphadoxine 500 mg and pyrimethamine 25 mg, and should *never* be given to anyone who is allergic to sulphonamides. Fatal epidermal necrolysis, syn. Lyell's syndrome, has occurred in two travellers with sulpha allergy who took Fansidar in urban Thailand, where there is no risk of malaria. Other adverse effects include haematopoietic abnormalities and skin rashes. None of the other drugs mentioned viz. Malarone (atovaquone/ proguanil), Maloprim (pyrimethamine/dapsone), Riamet (artemether/lumefantrine), or Euratesim™ (dihydroartemisinin/piperaquine) contain a sulphonamide.

29. A. All these three ACTs are effective against *P. falciparum* and are used in regular treatment as well as in SBET. Bioavailability is best with a fatty meal/drink when using Coartem™ and Riamet™ because of the lipid solubility of the lumefantrine moiety of these two drugs. Euratesim™ is water-soluble and need not be taken with a meal, fatty or otherwise. Since the PQP moiety of Euratesim™ has such a long half-life (24–34 days), this drug is also useful in preventing reinfection/ recrudescence of malaria. None is normally used against *P. vivax*.

30. A. Amodiaquine (Camoquin, Flavoquine) is a 4-aminoquinoline compound related to chloroquin and has both antimalarial and anti-inflammatory effects. It is useful in treating CRPF malaria and can be used as a weekly chemoprophylaxis. It is widely available in Africa. It clears parasitaemia less rapidly than Euratesim™. Like other ACTs (except Euratesim™) its bioavailability is significantly dependent on fat in the intestine. Dihydroartemisin is the least stable but probably the most active of the artemisinins.

31. A. Haeme is toxic to the blood stage of malarial parasites. Artemisinins appear to work by blocking the ability of the parasites to convert haeme into haemozoin. Qinghaosu (Chinese: 青蒿素) is a natural product derived from the wormwood plant (*Artemisia annua*). It was used in traditional Chinese medicine for many centuries as a treatment for malaria. Regular Chinese medicine finally recognized its value in the 1970s when it became apparent that quinghaosu and its derivatives surpassed all other medications in clearing falciparum parasitaemia. These derivatives were called artemisinins. One of the most popular among them was dihydroartemisinin (DHA). DHA is currently widely used in *P. falciparum* malaria. DHA is available both in oral and parenteral forms. A parenteral artemisinin plus mefloquine is generally a superior combination to quinine plus tetracycline in the treatment of severe cerebral malaria (unrousable coma).

32. D. ACT is the wisest choice. Euratesim (dihydroartemisinin/piperaquine phosphate, DHA/PQP 320/40 & 160/20) has been shown to exceed the 95% values for clinical and parasitological responses recommended by the WHO across Asia, Africa, and South America. This drug is also active against *P. vivax* malaria, although it was not originally marketed as such.

The short half-life of DHA (<2 hours) combined with the long half-life of PQP (3–4 weeks) not only allows for a rapid cure of malaria but also protects the patient from further attacks for at least a month. Furthermore, the simplicity of dosage, one tablet a day × 3 days, facilitates good compliance. PQP replaced chloroquin in 1978 in China because of its greater potency and tolerability. Avoid monotherapy for fear of inducing drug resistance.Other fixed combination ACTs, e.g. Riamet™ (arthemeter + lumefantrine), are not inferior but lack the long-acting piperaquine 'tail' of Euratesim™.

33. A. Malaria occurs in Afghanistan between May and November at altitudes below 2000 m. Proguanil 200 mg daily plus chloroquine base 310 mg weekly is the standard recommendation during this time. Doxycycline 100 mg daily or artovaquone/proguanil 250/100 are useful alternatives. In most instances only SBET is used. In all cases terminal prophylaxis with primaquine to destroy residual hypnozoites is strongly recommended. It is incumbent to have up-to-date information about the most suitable chemoprophylactic agent to give to any traveller.

Drugs in travellers' diarrhoea

1. D. Quinolone-resistant campylobacter is on the rise, especially in South-East Asia. Quinolone-resistant strains of S. typhi are also emerging. Normally double-strength co-trimoxazole (TMP-SMX) is used to treat Isospora belli and Cyclospora cayetanensis. While nitrazonaxide is the preferred drug in Cryptosporidium enteritis, other less effective agents are also used, e.g. atovaquone, azithromycin, metronidazole, paromomycin and co-trimoxazole. Crytosporidium is a cause of a profound watery diarrhoea and fever especially, but not exclusively, in AIDS patients.

2. Answers: A-4; B-1; C-3; D-2

3. B. ORS alone will only replace fluid loss but in many cases adding either azithromycin or a fluoroquinolone for 3 days is an effective treatment for dysentery. One does not use the two antibiotics together (option D).Loperamide (Imodium) and other antimotility agents such as bismuth subsalicylate (Pepto-Bismol) or diphenyoxylate (Lomotil) are contraindicated in dysentery or in diarrhoea with fever or severe abdominal pain.

4. D. Co-trimoxazole has given good results in diarrhoea due to Cyclospora cayetanensis. This protozoan was first reported by Ashford in 1979 but was not identifed until 1993. It is found worldwide and is associated with prolonged profuse watery diarrhoea often accompanied by fever. Humans seem to be the only host. The main source of infection is tap water, including chlorinated tap water. Faeco-oral transmission or animal-to-animal transmission does not appear to occur. Diagnosis involves finding oocysts in the stool and requires special techniques. Consider it when other causes have been outruled.

5. A. Loperamide is a safe and effective drug in treating non-specific TD. The usual dosage is 4 mg stat followed by 2 mg after each loose stool for up to 5 days (maximum 6–8 mg in 24 hours). It is not given to children under 4 years for fear of inducing colitis. It acts as both antimotility and antisecretory agent and therefore should not be given in dysentery (blood in stool) unless combined with an antibiotic. Loperamide is generally preferable to diphenyoxylate/atropine because of the anticholinergic (blurring of vision, tachycardia, urinary retention) and opiate effects (drowsiness, depression, confusion) of the latter.

6. A. The side effects of absorbed bismuth include benign blackening of the skin and mucous membranes. Blackened stools from the unabsorbed bismuth subsalicylate may mimic melaena. Tinnitus has also been reported. However, the most significant effects of absorbed bismuth are nephrotoxicity and CNS toxicity. Cases of bismuth-induced encephalopathy were reported in France, but the vast majority of people tolerate bismuth preparations well. Note that tinnitus is also associated with quinine and salicylates. In North America bismuth preparations are widely used to prevent and treat TD. A dose of two 600 mg tablets chewed four times a day reduces the number of stools passed by at least 50%. Bismuth should be considered as an alternative to antibiotics because it is safer and cheaper, and does not have the problem of antibiotic resistance. In the USA and Canada it is available over the counter but it is not readily available in Europe, Australia, or New Zealand.

7. D. The salicylates in both BSS and aspirin potentiate each other in causing adverse reactions. Reye's syndrome is a possibility in children and aggravation of viral infections, e.g. chicken pox, has also been reported. Unspecified adverse reactions include anxiety, confusion, depression, tinnitus, and weakness. Decreased absorption of many antibiotics occurs if they are taken within 6 hours of bismuth. Presumably the bivalent cations of bismuth lower the bioavailability of tetracycline. Bismuth is not approved for those <2 years of age.

8. D. Clean well-cooked food and good hygiene habits in both the kitchen and serving staff are paramount in the prophylaxis of TD. One may get TD even when eating in high-class hotels despite excellent personal hygiene.

9. C. Widespread use of any drug always creates the possibility of inducing resistance in microorganisms. In general one should not prescribe chemoprophylaxis against TD for those travelling overseas. Some exceptions can be made, e.g. where TD can ruin an important trip or where TD may aggravate an underlying medical condition (inflammatory bowel disease, HIV, diabetes mellitus). There is no clear evidence that prebiotics are useful in this regard.

10. C. Loperamide is the most effective. Kaolin helps to make stools more formed and is as good as BSS in reducing the number of stools passed, but neither is preferable to loperamide. Co-trimaxazole is probably underused in TD despite encountering growing resistance. Lomotil™ has limited antidiarrhoeal activity, is associated with unwanted anticholinergic effects and may cause central opiate depression, especially in children. In dysentery (fever, bloody stool) azithromycin is probably the drug of choice (1 g stat).

11. A. Skin patches can be used to deliver the heat-labile enterotoxin of ETEC. Such patches have been shown to reduce the severity of TD in humans and may have a promising future. Lactobacillus GG has a much better record in reducing TD than either *L. acidophilus* or *S. boulardii*. *Lactobacillus rhamnosus* GG was first isolated from the gastrointestinal tract of a healthy human being in 1983 and patented in 1985 by Gorbachand Goldini, hence the 'GG.' A report from Thailand showed that drinking tap water in two Thai cities was statistically protective. Perusal of the literature suggests that what one eats is of less importance in the genesis of TD than where one eats.

12. D. Rifaximin (Xifaxan™) is a semisynthetic antibiotic derived from rifamycin. Less than 3% is absorbed systemically and cross-resistance to either rifampicin or rifamycin does not appear to occur. It can be taken at any time, irrespective of food. The dose is 200 mg tid for 3 days. It is not used in dysentery.

13. D. Rifaximin is approved in 17 countries and has been used in Italy for over 25 years. It received approval from the FDA in May 2004. It probably does not interfere with OCs or with any drug metabolised by the human cytochrome P450 system. It is not used in children <12 years old although the manufacturers state that its 'safety and effectivnesss have not been tested in cildren under 2 years of age' which suggests it is safe to give from age 2 upwards. In contrast to macrolides it is ineffective against Campylobacter. Resistance to rifampicin is well documented and it is also been reported to cause immune haemolysis.

14. C. Rifaximin inhibits bacterial synthesis of ribonucleic acid and is active against many enteropathogens (Gram+, Gram–, aerobic, non-aerobic). It may also have some inhibitory effect against Cryptosporidium. However, it is currently only recommended against non-invasive strains of E. coli. We know that E. coli can develop resistance to rifaximin in vitro but we do not know if this has any clinical significance.

15. D. Some papers propose that rifaximin in doses of 500–600 mg daily for 14 days starting 72 hours before departure reduces the incidence of TD. Other papers suggest that placebo is just as good. It may be that in the groups studied personal food behaviour is influenced by the fact that the participants realized they were part of a clinical trial.

Miscellaneous

1. A. TMP-SMX, tetracyclines, and clarithromycin, e.g. Klacid™, are used in the treatment of *Mycoplasma pneumoniae*. This is important to know since *Mycoplasma pneumoniae* accounts for about 15% of all pneumonias and is easily spread by close contact, e.g. on cruise ships and package holidays. *Mycoplasma pneumoniae* is often insidious and atypical in presentation. TMP-SMX is also useful for treating melioidosis, cyclospora, and some cases of campylobacter. It is of little use in treating shigella, *S. typhi*, or myiasis. Resistance to TMP-SMX is now widespread.

2. A. Erythromycin is often the first choice antibiotic in Legionnaire's disease but TMP-SMX (co-trimoxazole) is a good alternative. Erythromycin is of little use in treating shigella or *S. typhi* and of no use in treating myiasis (diptera-fly larva infestation).

3. B. Mycoplasma can be treated by a variety of agents, including erythyromycin. *P. jirovecii* is treated—and prevented—by TMP-SMX. Pontiac fever is an acute flu-like illness that comes on a few hours after exposure to *L. pneumophila*. It needs no treatment and is only seen in the context of an epidemic of Legionnaire's disease.

4. Answers:

A-2. Artemisinins kill immature worms and have been used to prevent *S. japonicum*. Artemisinins are best known for their use in malaria. PZQ is the drug of choice in all cases of schistosomiasis.

B-4. Doyxcycline is known to kill the symbiotic wolbachia bacteria in filariasis and so is a useful adjunct to ivermectin. It is used to prevent malaria but never as a monotherapy because of its slow and relatively inefficient effect on parasitaemia and its failure to alleviate the clinical disease.

C-1, 2. Artemisinins combined with piperaquine or lumefantrine are the first-line treatment for malaria in most cases. Mefloquine is also a recognized treatment in the absence of ACT.

D-3. TMP-SMX (one double strength tablet bid × 7–10 days) is useful in many cases of TD due to Campylobacter. It is also useful in many cases of TD due to *Cyclospora cayetanensis* and *Isospora belli* as well as in a wide range of bacterial conditions in children where one is reluctant to give quinolones. Macrolide antibiotics (erythromycin and its semi-synthetic derivatives) are often helpful in Campylobacter infections. They are especially good in Thailand, where quinolone resistance now occurs in >50% of cases of Campylobacter diarrhoea.

5. A. PZQ as a stat dose of 40–60 mg/kg is deadly to adult worms and may be repeated after a few months if necessary. It should be taken with or shortly after a meal. Side effects are minimal, although disease exacerbation can be induced sometimes. Steroids may be given with PZQ in order to minimize any possible flare-up from reaction to the dying and dead worms. PZQ, 75 mg in a split dose, is used in some clinics (Christopher Hatz, personal communication).

The artemisinins have some antischistosomal effects, especially in Katayama fever, but their use is limited because of concerns about inducing malarial resistance.

6. C. Mefloquine alone (25 mg/kg) can reduce the worm load by >50% and when combined with artesunate appears to be a formidable agent against S. *haematobium*, especially in children. Artemisinin derivatives (artemeter, artesunate) are active against developing schistosomules.

PZQ is ineffective against young schistosomulae (up to 28 days old) but when given early does delay oviposition. This gives rise to the practice of giving artemisinin plus PZQ as an early post-exposure prophylaxis to non-immune travellers. Steroids will damp down severe allergic reactions, which can be very serious in some patients. None of these drugs affects cercarial penetration. See filariasis in chapter 14.

7. C. Loa loa is a filarial nematode that infests the rainforests of Central and West Africa. Humans contract it through the bite of a Chrysop fly (red fly, mango fly, horsefly, or deerfly). These are vicious and painful biters. Adult worms develop in subcutaneous tissue in 6–12 months and may live and reproduce there for >17 years. They produce millions of sheathed microfilariae seen typically during early afternoon in the peripheral blood. Transient red itchy swellings (Calabar swellings) may occur as a hypersensitive reaction to moving and damaged adult worms. Ivermectin, DEC, and albendazole can all be used to treat loa loa. Ivermectin paralyses the microflariae and prevents adult females producing any more. Like DEC, caution should be used when giving ivermectin if the mifcrofilaremia is >20,000/ml. Deaths have been reported after ivemectin in dual infections of loa loa and onchocerciasis. See Mazotti reaction and filariasis in chapter 14. Taeniasis and schistosomiasis are treated with PZQ.

8. A. Ivermectin as a single dose kills scabies mites. It is not licensed for this use in the USA at this time.

9. D. HAPE is characterized by a patchy pulmonary vasoconstriction with too little blood flow to some areas and too much to others. This patchy vasoconstriction is reversed by nifedipine, which blocks calcium channels and thereby relaxes the pulmonary vasculature. Other vasodilators are also useful, e.g. hydralazine, phentolamine, prostaglandins, nitric oxide, and sildenafil. Clearly a drug that dries the alveoli would be of immense help. Such therapy would be directed at stimulating the passage of Na^+ and H_2O from the alveoli into the alveolar epithelial cell and then inwards to the interstitial spaces, e.g. a drug that could activate Na/K/ATPase in the basolateral walls and the Na$^+$ channels in the luminal wall of the epithelial cells. Salmeterol, a β2-agonist, is of value in this regard since it increases alveolar fluid clearance.

Definitive treatment of HAPE is descent and oxygen therapy. Supplemental oxygen and the use of a portable hyperbaric chamber reduce help to reduce the pulmonary artery systolic pressure in such an emergency. Dexamethasone is often dramatic in relieving acute cerebral edema but less so in HAPE. See mountain climbing in chapter 10.

10. B. Photosensitivity implies an excess photoactivation with an unwanted cutaneous reaction from exposure to light. There are two types, photoallergic and phototoxic. Chemical photoallergic reactions occur when sunlight activates a topical drug so that it enters the skin and causes a local dermatitis, usually confined to the exposed areas. Chemical phototoxicity occurs when sunlight affects the drug (oral or topical) so that it provokes an antibody response and causes a dermatitis that may occur locally or all over the body. Photoallergic responses to a drug remain whenever there is re-exposure to that drug, phototoxic reactions recur when there is exposure to the sun even after the drug is long cleared. The distinction betweeen the two types is often blurred.

11. A. Doxycycline (a tetracycline) is a strong photosensitizer. Prolonged dosage of 100 mg per day probably sensitizes up to 3% of users. A sunscreen of high SPF (at least 20) should be used by those who are exposed to the sun a great deal, e.g. sunbathers and skiers. The photosensitization of cyclines is dose dependent and mainly triggered by UVB. Even photo-oncholysis has been reported in a traveller who used doxycycline. Other drugs that cause photosensitivity include thiazides, chlorpromazine, sulphonamides, nalidixic acid and proptryptiline.

12. A. Miltefosine (phosphochlorine analog) is the first effective oral drug for leishmaniasis. Although it was used initially in the treatment of cancer, its potential to treat leishmaniasis was pursued by Indian scientists who found cure rates of 98% in patients with visceral leishmaniasis. Similar cure rates were later reported from Colombia in patints with cutaneous leishmaniasis. Miltefosine has few adverse side effects, does not require refrigeration for storage, and has been used successfully to treat cases resistant to conventional antimony therapy. It is of no value in preventing malaria, TD, or MDRTB.

1. **Which of the following must be reported to the WHO by national governments according to international health regulations?**
    A. Leprosy
    B. HIV/AIDS
    C. Yellow fever
    D. Meningitis W-135

2. **How long must a second and subsequent yellow fever vaccination be given before entering a yellow fever area in order to be valid?**
    A. 10 days
    B. 4 days
    C. 1 day
    D. Any time right up to entry

3. **The most frequent cause of infectious death among travellers is**
    A. Respiratory tract infection
    B. Dengue
    C. Malaria
    D. Acute HIV

4. **Where is the most likely place in which to contract typhoid?**
    A. Brazil
    B. Egypt
    C. Nigeria
    D. India

5. **The concurrent administration of which of the following pairs of vaccines and medications may result in a reduced efficacy of the vaccine?**
    A. Yellow fever vaccine and mefloquine
    B. Japanese encephalitis vaccine and parenteral polio vaccine
    C. Oral typhoid vaccine and ciprofloxacin
    D. Oral polio and doxycycline

6. **Rabies vaccine**
   A. Is an inactivated viral vaccine
   B. Major brands are not interchangeable during the primary course
   C. Provides up to 3 months protection after 2 doses
   D. Should not be given to children under 2 years of age

7. **Hepatitis B**
   A. Is usually contracted by the faeco-oral route
   B. Is less transmissible than HIV
   C. Is a common cause of cancer of the liver
   D. Is usually associated with hepatitis E

8. **In immunodeficient or immunocompromised persons**
   A. Give a smaller dose of vaccine than usual
   B. Give a larger dose of vaccine than usual
   C. Avoid all vaccines
   D. Avoid recombinant vaccines

9. **A 30-year-old male traveller plans to travel widely in Egypt in August for 4 weeks, leaving on 2 August. He has had no previous travel vaccines. You see him on 29 July. Which of the following is the most important and appropriate single vaccine you would recommend?**
   A. Hepatitis B
   B. Typhoid
   C. Rabies
   D. Hepatitis A

10 **A 30-year-old male traveller plans to hike in the Atlas Mountains in Morocco, leaving on 2 August. He sees you on 29 July. Which of the following is the most important and appropriate single vaccine you would recommend?**
   A. Meningitis
   B. Diphtheria/tetanus
   C. Tick-borne encephalitis
   D. Hepatitis A

11. **IPV given by injection**
   A. Is less antigenic than OPV
   B. Can be given to travelling infants within a few days of birth
   C. Is the only form of polio vaccine that should be used
   D. Is now almost as cheap as OPV

12. Yellow fever vaccination in children

A. Is absolutely contraindicated in children <12 months
B. Is unnecessary in a breast-fed infant where the mother has had yellow fever vaccination within the previous 10 years
C. Is linked to encephalitis in young children
D. Requires a booster at 5 rather than 10 years to be effective

13. BCG

A. Is an inactivated viral vaccine
B. Is a conjugate vaccine
C. Is a recombinant vaccine derived from *M. bovis*
D. May confer protection against extra-pulmonary tuberculosis and miliary TB in infants less than 1 year old

14. Dengue fever

A. Is transmitted by the bite of a tick
B. Is transmitted by the bite of a mosquito
C. Is primarily a rural disease
D. Can now be acquired by travellers to Scandinavian countries

15. The most common adverse effect of chloroquine is

A. Stomach upsets
B. Interference with oral contraceptives
C. Haemolysis
D. Cataract

16. The blood picture in acute falciparum malaria includes

A. Marked eosinophilia
B. A rise in blood platelets
C. A significant lymphocytosis
D. Hypoglycaemia

17. TD in developing countries

A. Is usually due to salmonella and/or shigella
B. Is unlikely to occur if the traveller stays in five-star hotels
C. Is more likely in those who chose their own meals rather than in those who travel as part of an all-inclusive package
D. Usually occurs within the first 2 weeks of travel

18. TD due to quinolone-resistant Campylobacter is most common in which of the following countries?

A. Thailand
B. Peru
C. India
D. Mexico

SELF-TEST | **QUESTIONS** 239

19. In typhoid fever

A. The WIDAL test is still the gold standard for diagnosis
B. Culture of bone marrow aspirate gives a good recovery rate for *S. typhi*
C. The incubation period is usually less than a week
D. *S. typhi* is destroyed by gastric acid

20. At cruising altitude modern commercial aircraft are pressurized to

A. Sea level (760 mmHg)
B. 1000 feet
C. 8000 feet
D. 10,000 feet

21. The anopheles mosquito is recognized

A. By resting in a bottom-up posture
B. By being a larger mosquito than others
C. By having distinctive white spots on its wings
D. By having lateral floats attached to its thorax

22. Mosquitoes are attracted by

A. Sweat
B. A hairy skin
C. Leather watchstraps
D. The subject lying still

23. White water rafting is mostly associated with

A. Melioidosis
B. Anthrax
C. Legionella
D. Leptospirosis

24. The best way to make water potable is to

A. Boil it
B. Filter it
C. Treat it with organochlorines
D. Subject it to ultraviolet light

25. Air travel is contraindicated if the traveller has

A. An untreated compound fracture
B. PaO_2 less than 80 mmHg
C. Recent pneumothorax
D. A myocardial infarct within the previous 6 months

Answers on page 242.

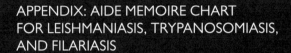

Disease	Where (most common)	Organism	Vector	Clinical	Treat
LEISHMANIASIS (a protozoon of genus Leishmania with kinetoplast and single flagellum; Related to trypanosomatids)					
Visceral (kala azar) VL	90% Indian subcontinent, Pockets Brazil, Sudan & middle East	*L.donovani complex L. tropica* (Old World)	Sandflies[1] (Phlebotominae) carry all types	Nil to low-grade fever to massive Hepatosplenomegaly	Antimonials Miltefosine Pentamidine
Cutaneous CL	90% Brazil, Peru, Middle East	*L. amazonis* (New World) Also *L. donovani, L. chagasi* etc		CL, ML, LR Persistent skin or mucosal ulcers/ lesions. ML is very disfiguring.	Miltefosine keto-, itra- & flu-conazole
Mucosal ML	90% Brazil, Bolivia, Peru			(Espundia). Damage & duration depends on species of organism	*Note mutual enhancement between Leishmaniasis and HIV*
Recidivans LR	Iran, Iraq	Usually *L. tropica.* Do not confuse with PKDL		Persistent recurrence of apparently healed skin lesions, like lupus vulgaris	
TRYPANOSOMIASIS (flagellated one-celled parasitic protozoon)					
Sleeping Sickness	East Africa	*T. rhodesiense*	Tsetse Fly	Fever, joint pain, Winterbottom's sign[2] Cerebral function	Melarsoprol (arsenic based)
	West Africa	*T. gambiense*	Tsetse Fly	finally deteriorates. Kerandel's sign[3]	Suramin
Chagas Disease	South and Central America	*T. cruzi*	Triatomine (kissing) reduviid bug	Acute: Cutaneous oedema, chagoma, Romana's sign[4] Chronic: megacolon cardiomyopathy, mega-oesophagus	Benznidazole Nifurtimox

FILARIASIS (filarial worm, nematode)

Lymphatic*	30% Africa	*W. Bancrofti*	Mosquitoes carry all types e.g. *Anopheles, Culex, Aedes Mansonia*	Nil to acute (adenolymphangitis, fever, TPE) to chronic (elephantiasis)	Ivermectin DEC Albendazole Doxycycline
	60% Indian subcontinent	*B. Malayi* *B. Timori*	*Culex quinquefasciatus* esp. in Asia & S America.	Brugian filariasis is generally a milder condition than bancroftian.	
	5% Far East	*W. Bancrofti & B. Malayi*			
	5% South/ Central America	*W. Bancrofti & B. Malayi*			
Onchocerciasis *The 'itch worm'*	Mostly sub-Saharan Africa	*O. volvulus*	Black fly (Simulium)	intense itch, subcut nodules, leopard skin	Ivermectin Doxycycline
Loiasis 'the eye worm'	West Africa	*Loa Loa*	Red Fly (Chrysops)	Calabar swellings Migrating adults, e.g. across eye	DEC Ivermectin

DEC diethycarbamazine. TPE tropical pulmonary eosinophilia. O. *onchocerca*, W. *wuchereria*; B. *brugia*. PKDL post-kala-azar dermal leishmaniasis.

[1] Phlebotominae are unable to bite through clothing

[2] Winterbottom's sign: lympahadenopathy most prominent in posterior triangle of neck

[3] Kerandel's sign: delayed hyperesthesia

[4] Romana's sign: unilateral orbital oedema often seen in early Chagas disease *75 million infected with *W. Bancrofti*, 6 million infected with *B. malayi* and *B. timori*.

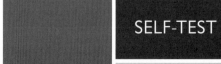

1-C; 2-D; 3-C; 4-D; 5-C; 6-A; 7-C; 8-B; 9-D; 10-D; 11-A; 12-C; 13-D; 14-B; 15-A; 16-D; 17-D; 18-A; 19-B; 20-C; 21-A; 22-A; 23-D; 24-A; 25-C

Key: ■ denotes question, ■ denotes answer